AF892436

Endothelial Dysfunction - A Novel Paradigm

Edited by Alaeddin Abukabda and Christopher Fonner

Published in London, United Kingdom

Endothelial Dysfunction - A Novel Paradigm
http://dx.doi.org/10.5772/intechopen.100929
Edited by Alaeddin Abukabda and Christopher Fonner

Contributors
Erjan Fikri, Ahmad Razi Maulana Alnaz, Fini Meirisa Alnaz, Anushree Gupta, Fernando Grover Páez, Javier Esparza Pimentel, Iwona Irena Wybranska, Yunhui Du, Yanru Duan, Shihan Zhang

© The Editor(s) and the Author(s) 2023
The rights of the editor(s) and the author(s) have been asserted in accordance with the Copyright, Designs and Patents Act 1988. All rights to the book as a whole are reserved by INTECHOPEN LIMITED. The book as a whole (compilation) cannot be reproduced, distributed or used for commercial or non-commercial purposes without INTECHOPEN LIMITED's written permission. Enquiries concerning the use of the book should be directed to INTECHOPEN LIMITED rights and permissions department (permissions@intechopen.com).
Violations are liable to prosecution under the governing Copyright Law.

Individual chapters of this publication are distributed under the terms of the Creative Commons Attribution 3.0 Unported License which permits commercial use, distribution and reproduction of the individual chapters, provided the original author(s) and source publication are appropriately acknowledged. If so indicated, certain images may not be included under the Creative Commons license. In such cases users will need to obtain permission from the license holder to reproduce the material. More details and guidelines concerning content reuse and adaptation can be found at http://www.intechopen.com/copyright-policy.html.

Notice
Statements and opinions expressed in the chapters are these of the individual contributors and not necessarily those of the editors or publisher. No responsibility is accepted for the accuracy of information contained in the published chapters. The publisher assumes no responsibility for any damage or injury to persons or property arising out of the use of any materials, instructions, methods or ideas contained in the book.

First published in London, United Kingdom, 2023 by IntechOpen
IntechOpen is the global imprint of INTECHOPEN LIMITED, registered in England and Wales, registration number: 11086078, 5 Princes Gate Court, London, SW7 2QJ, United Kingdom

British Library Cataloguing-in-Publication Data
A catalogue record for this book is available from the British Library

Additional hard and PDF copies can be obtained from orders@intechopen.com

Endothelial Dysfunction - A Novel Paradigm
Edited by Alaeddin Abukabda and Christopher Fonner
p. cm.
Print ISBN 978-1-80356-626-9
Online ISBN 978-1-80356-627-6
eBook (PDF) ISBN 978-1-80356-628-3

We are IntechOpen, the world's leading publisher of Open Access books

Built by scientists, for scientists

6,300+
Open access books available

170,000+
International authors and editors

190M+
Downloads

156
Countries delivered to

Our authors are among the
Top 1%
most cited scientists

12.2%
Contributors from top 500 universities

WEB OF SCIENCE™

Selection of our books indexed in the Book Citation Index in Web of Science™ Core Collection (BKCI)

Interested in publishing with us?
Contact book.department@intechopen.com

Numbers displayed above are based on latest data collected.
For more information visit www.intechopen.com

Meet the editors

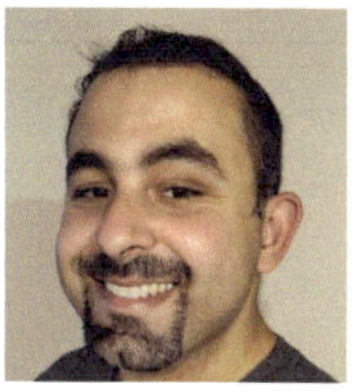

Dr. Abukabda graduated from Al Fateh Dental College, Libya, in 2007. He obtained a master's degree in Molecular Biology from Clarion University, USA, in 2011. He later obtained a Ph.D. in Cellular and Integrative Physiology from West Virginia University, USA, in 2018, and a Certification in Biostatistics from the School of Public Health at WVU. In 2018, he worked as a postdoctoral research associate at the Vascular Medicine Institute, University of Pittsburgh, USA. He has published and presented many articles on immunology, toxicology, and cardiovascular physiology. He serves as a reviewer for several journals. Dr. Abukabda is an Assistant Professor of Physiology at Lake Erie College of Osteopathic Medicine (LECOM), USA.

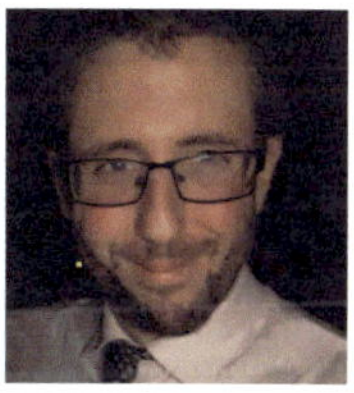

Dr. Christopher Fonner is an Associate Professor of Physiology at the Lake Erie College of Osteopathic Medicine (LECOM), USA. He teaches physiology to first-year medical school students as well as to graduate students in the MMS and Ph.D. programs. Dr. Fonner received his BSc in Biology from Gannon University, USA, in 2009, and a Ph.D. in Biology from Duquesne University, USA, in 2015. During his tenure at Duquesne, he served as a teaching assistant for several courses, including anatomy and physiology, general biology, mammalian physiology, physiology and molecular techniques for PT, and cell and systems physiology. From 2015 to 2019, Dr. Fonner was an Assistant Professor of Biology at Thiel College, USA, where he also served as the department chair of biology during 2018–2019. During his time at Thiel College, he instructed several courses, including human physiology, human anatomy, animal physiology, the physiological basis of exercise and physical fitness, introduction to exercise science, developmental biology, and foundations of biology. He also instructed several seminar courses, including a junior research seminar course and a senior seminar in biology. In addition to course instruction, Dr. Fonner served as an advisor to several student organizations, including the Tri-Beta Biological Honors Society and the Health Professions Institute, among others. Additionally, Dr. Fonner has served on numerous committees and has supervised several major undergraduate research projects. Dr. Fonner's research focuses primarily on three areas. His doctoral work involved the examination of behavioral and endocrinological responses to different stressors in amphibians. His current areas of interest include the examination of physiological responses to stressful stimuli in undergraduate and medical school students, as well as the use of technological and virtual simulation software in enhancing the understanding of various complex scientific concepts. If students are interested in any of these areas of research, they are encouraged to contact Dr. Fonner via e-mail. Dr. Fonner also has a considerable interest in scientific outreach and education. Previously, he coordinated and functioned as a group leader for various STEM-centered science outreach programs, both at Duquesne University and Thiel College.

Contents

Preface

The endothelium is a thin layer of cells that lines the inside of the heart and blood vessels. It is a fundamental determinant of cardiovascular health and its pathophysiological role has recently come under intense scrutiny.

This book presents novel aspects of endothelial dysfunction and provides a clinical context for them. It describes the molecular biology and genetics of endothelial dysfunction with a focus on potential therapeutic targets. It also discusses novel pathways associated with endothelial dysfunction and provides a real-world clinical correlate to emphasize the importance of understanding and managing endothelial dysfunction.

Alaeddin Abukabda
Assistant Professor of Physiology,
Lake Erie College of Osteopathic Medicine,
Erie, USA

Christopher Fonner
Associate Professor of Physiology,
Lake Erie College of Osteopathic Medicine,
Erie, USA

Section 1

Molecular Biology and Genetics of Endothelial Dysfunction

Chapter 1

Endothelial Dysfunction, Molecular Biology, Physiopathology, Diagnosis, and Treatment

Fernando Grover Páez and Javier Esparza Pimentel

Abstract

Endothelial cell dysfunction has lately become one of the principal subjects being incorporated into the assessment of cardiovascular risk because of the relevance that has been shown in several clinical studies. Comprehending and incorporating basic physiological knowledge, about endothelium molecular biology and vascular tonicity, is key to understanding the relevance of this topic. The approach of endothelial dysfunction physiopathology is overly complex and widely studied, but it can be enrolled into both consumption of bioavailable NO and deficit production of NO. In the last decades, scientific equipment has been developed from the necessity of creating non-invasive tools to measure arterial stiffness, being FMD one of the first and most used ones. Once the endothelial cell dysfunction was identified, several drugs and bioactive substances were evaluated because of their potential to decrease the level of arterial stiffness and improve life quality, such as polyphenols, phosphodiesterase five inhibitors, and new incoming therapies.

Keywords: endothelial cell dysfunction, nitric oxide, flow mediated dilatation, polyphenols, PDE5i

1. Introduction

Endothelial cell dysfunction (ECD) is defined as an altered metabolism of available nitric oxide (NO), or an imbalance of relaxing and constrictor endothelial factors [1]. Many of the physiological functions of the endothelial cells (ECs) are involved with the regulation of vascular tonicity, balancing of blood fluidity and thrombosis through coagulation and fibrinolysis factors, vascular inflammatory and immunological process control, and several growth factors [2]. Any alteration in these systems can lead to a loss of vascular homeostasis and contribute to developing endothelial dysfunction [1, 2].

2. Endothelium molecular biology, vascular tonicity and its regulation

Vascular tonicity is regulated by multiple molecules, proteins, hormones, and peptides secreted or with action mechanisms on the ECs such as an atrial natriuretic peptide, eicosanoids, adrenal steroids, sodium, and water excretion, and reno-medullary endothelial systems [3].

Examples of several endothelium-derived hyperpolarizing factors are NO and prostacyclin, whereas endothelin-1 (ET-1), angiotensin II, thromboxane A2 and reactive oxygen species (ROS), relaxing factors [4].

2.1 Nitric oxide (NO)

NO is a reactive, diffusible gaseous free radical whit strong intrinsic oxidant properties. It is produced locally at ECs by three different isoforms of NO synthase (NOS) enzymes, each with unique expression and functional properties: neuronal NOS (nNOS, NOS1), inducible NOS (iNOS, NOS2), and endothelial NOS (eNOS, NOS3) [5].

Elevated levels of intracellular Ca2+, acting through calmodulin, activates nNOS and eNOS respectively; iNOS is less susceptible to Ca2+, but around 1000 times more inducible by inflammatory stimuli such as TNF- α, IL-1β, and IFN-γ [6]. The NOS produced NO by catalyzing the oxidation of the nitrogen guanide of the L-arginine and O^2 producing L-citrulline and NO (**Figure 1**) [5, 6]. The NO activates soluble guanylyl cyclase (sGC), which at binding creates an augmentation of the Vmax of sGC and, consequently, rising the cellular cyclic guanosine monophosphate (cGMP) [6].

The cGMP vascular effects are mediated by several mechanisms, being the activation of protein kinase G (PKG) one of the main processes, conducting vasodilatation by means of release inhibition of Ca2+ mediated by inositol 1,4,5-trisphosphate (IP3) [6].

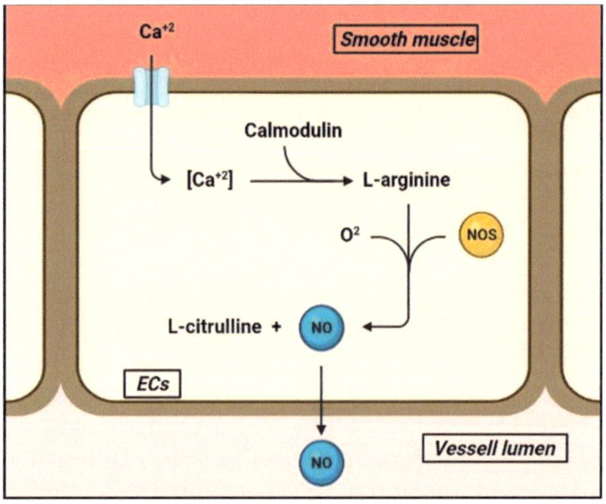

Figure 1.
The graphic shows the activation of NOS mediated by Calmodulin/Ca^{+2}. Subsequently, NOS produced NO and L-citrulline starting from L-arginine and O^2. Original graphic created with BioRender.com.

2.2 Endothelin-1 (ET-1)

ET-1 is a peptide of 21 amino acids that has two disulfide junctions, synthesized from a 39 amino acid precursor sequence named pre-pro endothelin by the activity of endothelin-converting enzyme (ECE) (**Figure 2**). ECE-1 restricts the synthesis of ET-1. The ET-1 its produced mainly in ECs, induced by several cytokines, angiotensin II and mechanical stress. It is codified by EDN1 gene, which expression is reduced by NO and prostaglandin I2 [7].

There are two basic types of ET-1 receptors: ETA and ETB. Both receptors are coupled to a G-protein and to the formation of IP3. ETA is, in normal conditions, the most prevalent of these ET-1 receptors [8].

ET-1 action is characterized by vasoconstriction; this effect is initiated once it binds to ETA receptor. The union of these results in the activation of Gq-PLC-IP3 pathway. IP3 induces the release of Ca2+ of the endoplasmic reticule by opening the L-type Ca2+ channels and increasing the cytosolic Ca2+, which produced the contraction of the muscular smooth cells and subsequent vasoconstriction (**Figure 3**) [1, 7, 8].

Despite the presence of ETB receptor on vascular smooth cells, it is also found on ECs, which stimulates the formation of NO causing vasodilatation, and additionally decreases the ET-1 synthesis causing relaxation [1].

3. Endothelial dysfunction physiopathology

ECD is defined biochemically by a decreased amount of available NO in the vasculature. There are multiple mechanisms that reduce this value, moreover, the whole dysfunction can be enrolled into two main categories [9].

3.1 Consumption of bioavailable NO

Altered NO metabolism due to elevated degradation of NO, inactivation of NO, or presence of NO inhibitors may be due to the elevation in oxidative stress [10]. NO is a highly diffusible and reactive species with an unpaired electron, because of this, there are a variety of chemical components that impede appropriate signaling [11]. Some of the principal agents of this deficiency are ROS and superoxide (O^{2-}).

ROS increases the activity of stimulants such as inflammation, radiation, advanced age, obesity, and sundry chemical substances. Superoxide is an important

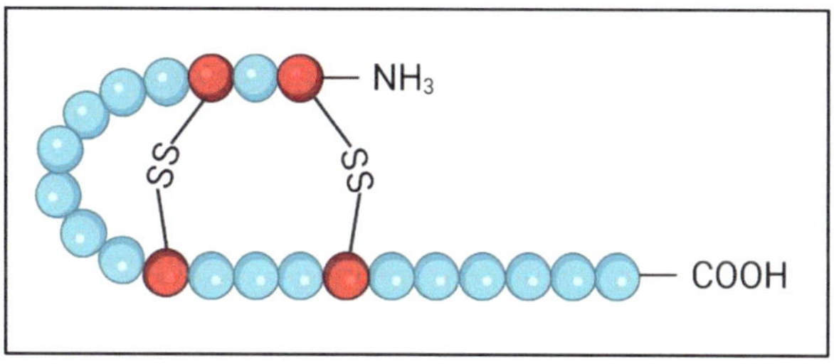

Figure 2.
Amino acid sequence of ET1, characterized by the presence of 21 amino acids and two disulfide junctions. Original graphic created with BioRender.com.

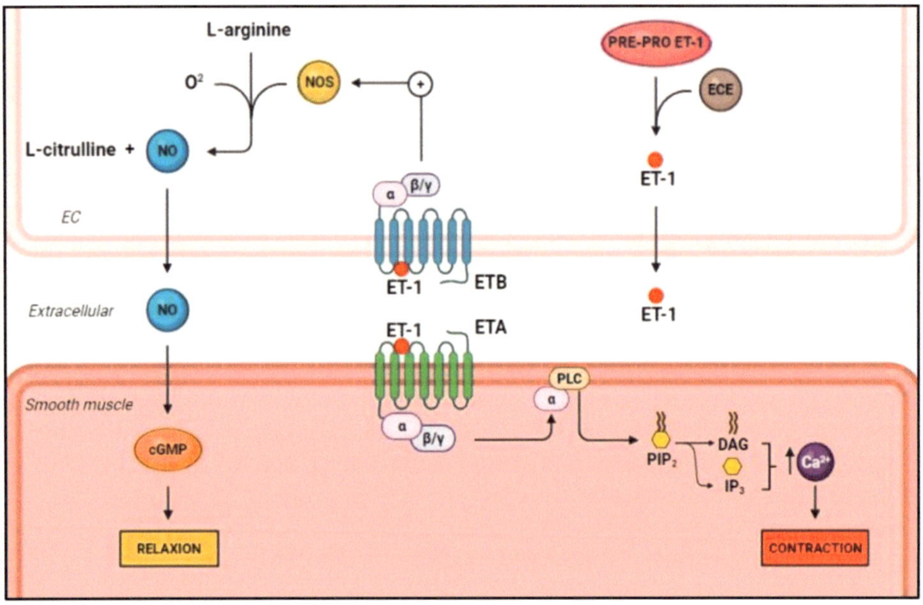

Figure 3.
The ET-1, synthesized from pre-pro ET1 by the activity of ECE in ECs, binds to ETA receptor in vascular smooth muscle and activates the pathway Gq-PLC-IP3, which rises cytosolic Ca2+ and induces muscular contraction. ET-1 can also activate ETB receptor in ECs leading to an increase in NOS activity and augmentation of bioavailable NO. Original graphic created with BioRender.com.

radical for cardiovascular biology, formed by one-electron reduction of oxygen. At a cellular level, increase oxidative stress causes damage by altering several molecules' structures like deoxyribonucleic acid, proteins, lipids, and carbohydrates [12].

3.2 Deficit production of NO

Approaching ECD through the deficit of NO production, modifications of eNOS is one of the processes that stand out in this category, being eNOS uncoupling is a major mechanism. This enzyme requires dimerization in the presence of heme and BH4 for an effective electron movement to L-arginine and the subsequent formation of NO and L-citrulline [3, 4, 13]. When this relation is disrupted, the outcome is that eNOS function as a weak NADPH oxidase, generating O^{2-} instead of NO, a process denominated eNOS uncoupling. Several mechanisms induce eNOS uncoupling, which increases local oxidative stress and removes the vasodilatation effect of NO [13].

Many pathways contribute to eNOS uncoupling, being ONOO one of the main. Also known as peroxynitrite, ONOO is an oxidant and nitrating agent with an unstable structural isomer of nitrate. The formation of this molecule is due to the reaction of free radical superoxide, with free radical nitric oxide. ONOO disrupts a zinc-thiolate cluster in eNOS and oxidizes BH4 to BH3, both creating an eNOS uncoupling and creating a cycle of ROS production [14].

Other, but also well-known, mechanism is L-arginine decrease associated with its inhibitor asymmetric dimethyl-L-arginine (ADMA). ADMA is an endogenous protein produced by N-methyltransferase type 1, elevated in redox status, and degraded by dimethylarginine dimethylaminohydrolase, altered by oxidative stress [15, 16].

DOI: http://dx.doi.org/10.5772/intechopen.107481

4. Diagnosis

Cardiovascular disease (CVD) remains as the principal cause of morbidity and mortality worldwide [17]. During last century multiples, studies have been developed with the intention to identify the association between several lifestyle factors and the probability of suffering CVD [18]. Moreover, it is established the presence of cardiovascular risk factors (CVRF) in early childhood is a predictor of CVD in their lifetime [18, 19].

At the end of the last century, some equipments were created and able to identify the endothelium condition through non-invasive tools. Flow-mediated dilation (FMD) has become the most popular and widely used method for examining noninvasive peripheral artery endothelium-dependent dilation [20].

4.1 FMD

Flow-mediated dilation represents an endothelium-dependent, largely NO-mediated dilatation of conduit arteries in response to an imposed increase in blood flow and shear stress first described in 1992 [20].

4.1.1 FMD procedure

FMD is typically assessed in brachial artery with a standardized diameter of 3–5 mm. Through a high-resolution B-mode ultrasound, images of the brachial artery are taken, usually with an ultrasound probe of 7.5–12 MHz [21]. An approach by tangential scanning is a common mistake and results in underestimation of the true brachial artery diameter (**Figure 4**). Recent studies, which adopt H-shaped, probe capturing two short-axis and one long-axis for automatic probe position correction may overcome this previous limitation [22].

A simultaneous evaluation of pulse-wave Doppler velocity is recommended, given the importance of shear stress as the eliciting stimulus for dilatation. The recommended isonation angle is <60° for optimal data acquisition, which should be kept constant [23, 24].

To ensure an optimal image throughout the hole FMD procedure, a probe-holding device is recommended. A stereotactic adjustable probe-holding device allows adjustment of probe position during the test, allowing to maintain the same scan in the study [25].

Many subject-related factors can influence FMD such as alcohol, smoking, food, supplements, drugs, physical activity, and mental stress. Some factors directly stimulated NO-release, but others, such as acute physical exercise and mental stress, modify baseline vasomotor tone [26, 27].

4.1.2 Clinical evidence

In a study, brachial FMD has associated whit intima-media thickness progression in a population free of CVD, and in hypertensive, postmenopausal women [28]. A follow-up study in hypertensive patients with FMD predicted target organ damage progression for 3 years, even adjusted for known CVRF [29].

One meta-analysis described a significant 8–13% lower risk of CVD per percentage point increase in brachial artery FMD (e.g. from 7–8% dilatation). This reduction

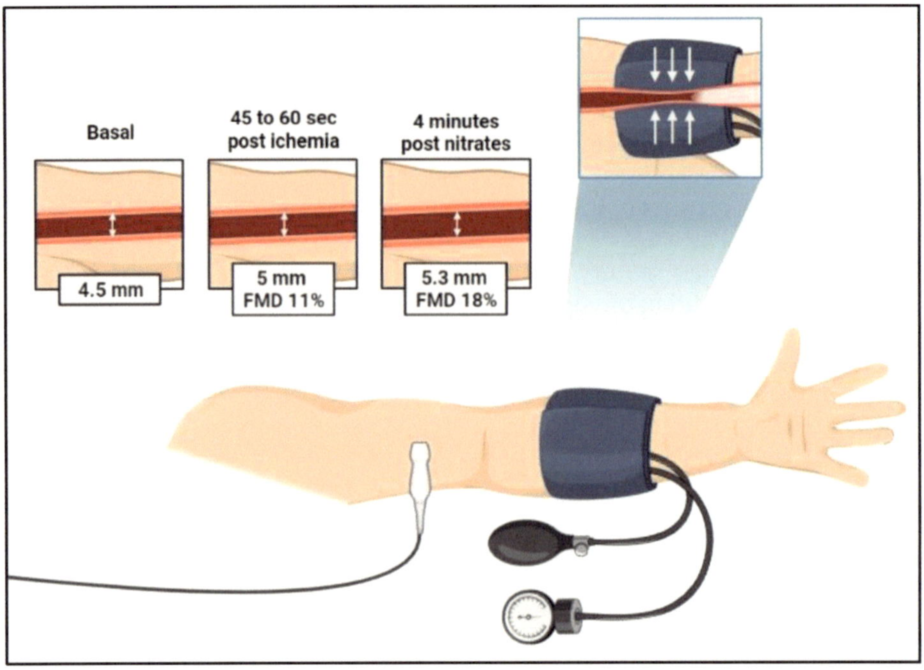

Figure 4.
FMD representation with cuff positioned in the forearm. Through ultrasound assessment, brachial artery diameter is measured before and 5 minutes after the ischemia. FMD can oscillate depending on if a hypertensive drug is used before the procedure such as nitrates. Original graphic created with BioRender.com.

was present in high and low-risk population but appeared larger in patients with established CVD [30, 31].

The clinical value of long-term changes in FMD may have a prognostic implication. For interventional trials FMD could represent a surrogate endpoint, especially since FMD is a tool with a rapid response effect to therapies, allowing recognition and identification of new bioactive substances or drugs able to modify FMD [32].

5. Treatment

5.1 Lifestyle

It is well established that lifestyle interventions have a main role in prevention of CVD. Many activities such as diet, aerobic exercise, quitting smoking and alcohol, and a non-sedentary day routine, have shown a significant reduction in blood pressure (BP) and arterial stiffness [33].

5.1.1 Mediterranean diet

The diet is one of the tractable modifiers of vascular health and BP, which has exhibited that targeting the whole diet has a more significant effect on BP than focusing on individual foods and nutrients [34].

The prevention with Mediterranean-style diet in several trials in patients with high CVRF showed that a Mediterranean diet supplemented with olive oil or nuts, reduced diastolic blood pressure by −1.5 mm Hg and − 0.7 mm Hg respectively, in comparison with low-fat diet over 4 years [35].

The recommendation to incorporate Mediterranean diet for older adults aiming its effect on BP and arterial stiffness is established in a 12-month randomized controlled trial called NU-AGE study. A total of 1294 healthy participants were included, aged 65 to 79 years, recruited from 5 European centers, and arterial stiffness was assessed in 225 participants using the Vicorder device measuring both carotid-femoral pulse wave velocity (PWV) and augmentation index (AIx) [36, 37]. The intervention group received individually tailored standardized dietary advice and commercially available foods to increase adherence to a Mediterranean diet, and the control group continued their habitual diet, and were provided with current national dietary guidance. Of the original sample, 1142 participants completed the trial, and after 1 year, the intervention group resulted in a significant reduction in systolic blood pressure (−5.5 mm Hg; 95% CI, −10.7 to −0.4; P = 0.03), and in a subset (n = 225), augmentation index was improved following intervention (−12.4; 95% CI, −24.4 to −0.5; P = 0.04), with no change in pulse wave velocity [37].

The favorable effects of the Mediterranean diet on health may result from high intake of omega-6 and omega-3 fatty acids, fibers, antioxidants, and polyphenols [38].

5.1.2 Polyphenols

There are scientific studies that showed polyphenol-enriched diet impedes hyperlipidemia and coronary endothelial dysfunction, both by counteracting vascular inflammation and oxidative damage by activating Akt/eNOS pathway [39]. Some of the polyphenol's effects are linked to the promotion of SIRT1-induced repression of the p38 MAPK/NF-kappaB pathway and ROS production [40].

When they come from virgin olive they reduce inflammatory angiogenesis in ECs through inhibition of matrix metalloproteinase-9 and cyclooxygenase-2, supporting the protective role of dietary polyphenols both in atherosclerosis and cancer [41].

5.2 Pharmacological therapy

Several drugs have actions mechanism involved in the physiological pathways of endothelial regulation and vascular tonicity, therefore this section will be discussed briefly a few of them.

5.2.1 PDE5i

Phosphodiesterase of cyclic nucleotide is a family of enzymes that hydrolyzed the cyclic nucleotides 3′-5′ to their 5′ monophophates analogs [42].

Vardenafil is one of many PDE5i in which a reduction of arterial stiffness has been reported. In one study twelve patients with erectile dysfunction, mean age of 58 ± 9 years, received verdanafil20 mg per day, in a randomized, placebo-controlled, double-blind2-way crossover design. Aortic stiffness was evaluated through carotid-femoral PWV and AIx. PWV decreased significantly (0.7 m/s, P = .001), denoting a decrease in aortic stiffness, and AIx decreased significantly (by 7%, P = .008), denoting a decreased effect of wave reflections from the periphery [43].

5.2.2 New therapies

Recent studies showed that microRNAs have a key role during atherosclerotic plaque formation, representing a potential new target for developing drugs.

In atherosclerotic plaque, miR-143 was found to be upregulated, and its overexpression in human umbilical vein endothelial cells (HUVECs) suppressed glycolysis by targeting hexokinase 2, leading to endothelial dysfunction [44]. And, in vivo, the inhibition of miR-92a, a regulator of endothelial proliferation and angiogenesis after ischemia, results in beneficial effects on the endothelium such as reducing inflammation and decreasing plaque size [45, 46].

Recent evidence shows several epigenetic pathways involved in endothelial dysfunction and related to cardiovascular diseases which will be discussed in the following.

Histone deacetylase 1 (HDAC1) overexpression in bovine aortic endothelial cells triggers a reduction of eNOS lysine acetylation and NO production. Its inhibition can stand as a therapy for preventing endothelial dysfunction. Additionally, HDAC1 decline leads to no change in eNOS acetylation, otherwise increasing basal nitrate NO formation [46, 47].

Another study evidence that resveratrol, a phenol produced naturally by different plants, prevents TNF-α-induced injury from damaging HUVECs by stimulating sirtuin-1 (SIRT1) and repressing p38 MAPK/NF-kappaB pathway and ROS production [40, 46].

Additionally, another NAD-dependent deacetylase, SIRT6 is expressed in atherosclerotic disease in human patients. In several mice studies, absence and haploinsufficient SIRT6 have been associated with monocyte adhesion to endothelium, augmentation of atherosclerosis gene expression, impaired vasorelaxation, and overexpression of VCAM-1 [48, 49]. Being so this knowledge is a potential subject for investigation of novel therapies counteracting atherosclerosis and decreasing endothelial dysfunction.

6. Conclusions

ECD is a vast, interesting, and shallow subject shortly explored by the scientific community, therefore, the actual information about this topic is very limited. Further clinical and molecular research should be addressed for a better understanding of the entire implications of these pathways in clinical and molecular investigations.

Moreover, current equipment for addressing clinical non-invasive parameters of arterial stiffness is emerging and earning a relevant place in cardiovascular risk assessment, therefore, these tools are already being incorporated in several international medical guidelines as an important parameter to consider.

Acknowledgements

We want to thank Aitana Rangel Garibay for editing this chapter.

Conflict of interest

There was no conflict of interest in the making of this document.

Appendices and nomenclature

ECD	Endothelial cell dysfunction
NO	Nitric oxide
ECs	Endothelial cells
ET-1	Endothelin-1
ROS	Reactive oxygen species
NOS	NO synthase
nNOS, NOS1	Neuronal NOS
iNOS, NOS2	Inducible NOS
eNOS, NOS3	Endothelial NOS
sGC	Soluble guanylyl cyclase
PKG	Protein kinase G
IP3	1,4,5-trisphosphate
ECE	Endothelin-converting enzyme
O^{2-}	Superoxide
CVD	Cardiovascular disease
CVRF	Cardiovascular risk factors
FMD	Flow mediated dilation
BP	Blood pressure
PWV	Pulse wave velocity
AIx	Augmentation index
PDE5i	Phosphodiesterase 5′ inhibitors
ADMA	Asymmetric dimethyl-L-arginine
HUVECs	Human umbilical vein endothelial cells
HDAC1	Histone deacetylase 1
SIRT1	Sirtuin-1

Author details

Fernando Grover Páez* and Javier Esparza Pimentel
University of Guadalajara, Vascular Mechanic of the Institute of Experimental and Clinical Therapeutics (INTEC), Guadalajara, Mexico

*Address all correspondence to: fgroverp@hotmail.com

IntechOpen

© 2022 The Author(s). Licensee IntechOpen. This chapter is distributed under the terms of the Creative Commons Attribution License (http://creativecommons.org/licenses/by/3.0), which permits unrestricted use, distribution, and reproduction in any medium, provided the original work is properly cited.

References

[1] Vanhoutte PM, Shimokawa H, Tang EH, Feletou M. Endothelial dysfunction and vascular disease. Acta Physiologica. 2009;**196**(2):193-222. DOI: 10.1111/j.1748-1716.2009.01964.x

[2] Chistiakov DA, Orekhov AN, Bobryshev YV. Endothelial barrier and its abnormalities in cardiovascular disease. Frontiers in Physiology. 2015;**6**:365. DOI: 10.3389/fphys.2015.00365

[3] Cahill PA, Redmond EM. Vascular endothelium. Gatekeeper of vessel health. Atherosclerosis. 2016;**248**:97-109. DOI: 10.1016/j.atherosclerosis.2016.03.007

[4] Dawes MG, Bartlett G, Coats AJ, Juszczak E. Comparing the effects of white coat hypertension and sustained hypertension on mortality in a UK primary care setting. The Annals of Family Medicine. 2008;**6**(5):390-396. DOI: 10.1370/afm.865

[5] Förstermann U, Sessa WC. Nitric oxide synthases: Regulation and function. European Heart Journal. 2012;**33**(7):829-837d. DOI: 10.1093/eurheartj/ehr304

[6] Tsai EJ, Kass DA. Cyclic GMP signaling in cardiovascular pathophysiology and therapeutics. Pharmacology Therapeutics. 2009;**122**(3):216-238. DOI: 10.1016/j.pharmthera.2009.02.009

[7] Davenport AP, Hyndman KA, Dhaun N, et al. Endothelin. Pharmacological Reviews. 2016;**68**(2):357-418. DOI: 10.1124/pr.115.011833

[8] Barton M. The discovery of endothelium-dependent contraction: The legacy of Paul M Vanhoutte. Pharmacological Research. 2011;**63**(6):455-462. DOI: 10.1016/j.phrs.2011.02.013

[9] Landmesser U, Dikalov S, Price SR, et al. Oxidation of tetrahydrobiopterin leads to uncoupling of endothelial cell nitric oxide synthase in hypertension. The Journal of Clinical Investigation. 2003;**111**(8):1201-1209. DOI: 10.1172/JCI14172

[10] Bonetti PO, Lerman LO, Lerman A. Endothelial dysfunction: A marker of atherosclerotic risk. Arteriosclerosis, Thrombosis, and Vascular Biology. 2003;**23**(2):168-175. DOI: 10.1161/01.atv.0000051384.43104.fc

[11] Pacher P, Beckman JS, Liaudet L. Nitric oxide and peroxynitrite in health and disease. Physiological Reviews. 2007;**87**(1):315-424. DOI: 10.1152/physrev.00029.2006

[12] González J, Valls N, Brito R, Rodrigo R. Essential hypertension and oxidative stress: New insights. World Journal of Cardiology. 2014;**6**(6):353-366. DOI: 10.4330/wjc.v6.i6.353

[13] Kuzkaya N, Weissmann N, Harrison DG, Dikalov S. Interactions of peroxynitrite, tetrahydrobiopterin, ascorbic acid, and thiols: Implications for uncoupling endothelial nitric-oxide synthase. Journal of Biological Chemistry. 2003;**278**(25):22546-22554. DOI: 10.1074/jbc.M302227200

[14] Aicher A, Heeschen C, Mildner-Rihm C, et al. Essential role of endothelial nitric oxide synthase for mobilization of stem and progenitor cells. [published correction appears in Nat Med. 2004 Sep;10(9):999. Nature

Medicine. 2003;**9**(11):1370-1376. DOI: 10.1038/nm948

[15] Karbach S, Wenzel P, Waisman A, Munzel T, Daiber A. eNOS uncoupling in cardiovascular diseases--the role of oxidative stress and inflammation. Current Pharmaceutical Design. 2014;**20**(22):3579-3594. DOI: 10.2174/13816128113196660748

[16] Cyr AR, Huckaby LV, Shiva SS, Zuckerbraun BS. Nitric oxide and endothelial dysfunction. Critical Care Clinics. 2020;**36**(2):307-321. DOI: 10.1016/j.ccc.2019.12.009

[17] World Health Organization. WHO Mortality Database. Geneva, Switzerland: World Health Organization, Department of Health Statistics and Information Systems; 2019

[18] Sytkowski PA, Kannel WB, D'Agostino RB. Changes in risk factors and the decline in mortality from cardiovascular disease. The Framingham Heart Study. New England Journal of Medicine. 1990;**322**(23):1635-1641. DOI: 10.1056/NEJM199006073222304

[19] Berenson GS, Srinivasan SR, Bao W, Newman WP 3rd, Tracy RE, Wattigney WA. Association between multiple cardiovascular risk factors and atherosclerosis in children and young adults. The Bogalusa Heart Study. New England Journal of Medicine. 1998;**338**(23):1650-1656. DOI: 10.1056/NEJM199806043382302

[20] Celermajer DS, Sorensen KE, Gooch VM, et al. Non-invasive detection of endothelial dysfunction in children and adults at risk of atherosclerosis. Lancet. 1992;**340**(8828):1111-1115. DOI: 10.1016/0140-6736(92)93147-f

[21] Gemignani V, Faita F, Ghiadoni L, Poggianti E, Demi M. A system for real-time measurement of the brachial artery diameter in B-mode ultrasound images. IEEE Transactions on Medical Imaging. 2007;**26**(3):393-404. DOI: 10.1109/TMI.2006.891477

[22] Tomiyama H, Kohro T, Higashi Y, et al. Reliability of measurement of endothelial function across multiple institutions and establishment of reference values in Japanese. Atherosclerosis. 2015;**242**(2):433-442. DOI: 10.1016/j.atherosclerosis.2015.08.001

[23] Padilla J, Johnson BD, Newcomer SC, et al. Normalization of flow-mediated dilation to shear stress area under the curve eliminates the impact of variable hyperemic stimulus. Cardiovascular Ultrasound. 2008;6:44. Published 2008 Sep 4. DOI:10.1186/1476-7120-6-44

[24] Oates C, editor. Cardiovascular Haemodynamics and Doppler Waveforms Explained. Cambridge University Press; 2001

[25] Donald AE, Halcox JP, Charakida M, et al. Methodological approaches to optimize reproducibility and power in clinical studies of flow-mediated dilation. Journal of the American College of Cardiology. 2008;**51**(20):1959-1964. DOI: 10.1016/j.jacc.2008.02.044

[26] Thijssen DH, Black MA, Pyke KE, et al. Assessment of flow-mediated dilation in humans: A methodological and physiological guideline. American Journal of Physiology-Heart and Circulatory Physiology. 2011;**300**(1):H2-H12. DOI: 10.1152/ajpheart.00471.2010

[27] Dawson EA, Green DJ, Cable NT, Thijssen DH. Effects of acute exercise on flow-mediated dilatation in healthy humans. Journal of Applied Physiology. 2013;**115**(11):1589-1598. 1985. DOI: 10.1152/japplphysiol.00450.2013

[28] Rossi R, Nuzzo A, Olaru AI, Origliani G, Modena MG. Endothelial function affects early carotid atherosclerosis progression in hypertensive postmenopausal women. Journal of Hypertension. 2011;**29**(6):1136-1144. DOI: 10.1097/HJH.0b013e328345d950

[29] Yang Y, Xu JZ, Wang Y, Tang XF, Gao PJ. Brachial flow-mediated dilation predicts subclinical target organ damage progression in essential hypertensive patients: A 3-year follow-up study. Journal of Hypertension. 2014;**32**(12):2393-2400. DOI: 10.1097/HJH.0000000000000337

[30] Xu Y, Arora RC, Hiebert BM, et al. Non-invasive endothelial function testing and the risk of adverse outcomes: A systematic review and meta-analysis. European Heart Journal Cardiovascular Imaging. 2014;**15**(7):736-746. DOI: 10.1093/ehjci/jet256

[31] Inaba Y, Chen JA, Bergmann SR. Prediction of future cardiovascular outcomes by flow-mediated vasodilatation of brachial artery: A meta-analysis. The International Journal of Cardiovascular Imaging. 2010;**26**(6):631-640. DOI: 10.1007/s10554-010-9616-1

[32] Lüscher TF, Taddei S, Kaski JC, et al. Vascular effects and safety of dalcetrapib in patients with or at risk of coronary heart disease: The dal-VESSEL randomized clinical trial. European Heart Journal. 2012;**33**(7):857-865. DOI: 10.1093/eurheartj/ehs019

[33] Marin C, Ramirez R, Delgado-Lista J, et al. Mediterranean diet reduces endothelial damage and improves the regenerative capacity of endothelium. American Journal of Clinical Nutrition. 2011;**93**(2):267-274. DOI: 10.3945/ajcn.110.006866

[34] Appel LJ. Lifestyle modification as a means to prevent and treat high blood pressure. Journal of the American Society of Nephrology. 2003;**14**(7 Suppl. 2): S99-S102. DOI: 10.1097/01.asn.0000070141.69483.5a

[35] Toledo E, Hu FB, Estruch R, et al. Effect of the Mediterranean diet on blood pressure in the PREDIMED trial: Results from a randomized controlled trial. BMC Medicine. 2013;**11**:207. Published 2013 Sep 19. DOI: 10.1186/1741-7015-11-207

[36] Pucci G, Cheriyan J, Hubsch A, et al. Evaluation of the Vicorder, a novel cuff-based device for the noninvasive estimation of central blood pressure. Journal of Hypertension. 2013;**31**(1):77-85. DOI: 10.1097/HJH.0b013e32835a8eb1

[37] Jennings A, Berendsen AM, de Groot LCPGM, et al. Mediterranean-style diet improves systolic blood pressure and arterial stiffness in older adults. Hypertension. 2019;**73**(3):578-586. DOI: 10.1161/hypertensionaha.118.12259

[38] Zamora-Ros R, Serafini M, Estruch R, et al. Mediterranean diet and non enzymatic antioxidant capacity in the PREDIMED study: Evidence for a mechanism of antioxidant tuning. Nutrition, Metabolism, and Cardiovascular Diseases. 2013;**23**(12):1167-1174. DOI: 10.1016/j.numecd.2012.12.008

[39] Vilahur G, Padró T, Casaní L, et al. Polyphenol-enriched diet prevents coronary endothelial dysfunction by activating the Akt/eNOS pathway. Revista Espanola de Cardiologia. 2015;**68**(3):216-225. DOI: 10.1016/j.rec.2014.04.021

[40] Pan W, Yu H, Huang S, Zhu P. Resveratrol protects against TNF-α-induced injury in human umbilical endothelial cells through promoting

sirtuin-1-induced repression of NF-KB and p38 MAPK. PLoS One. 2016;**11**(1):e0147034. DOI: 10.1371/journal.pone.0147034

[41] Scoditti E, Calabriso N, Massaro M, et al. Mediterranean diet polyphenols reduce inflammatory angiogenesis through MMP-9 and COX-2 inhibition in human vascular endothelial cells: A potentially protective mechanism in atherosclerotic vascular disease and cancer. Archives of Biochemistry and Biophysics. 2012;**527**(2):81-89. DOI: 10.1016/j.abb.2012.05.003

[42] Omori K, Kotera J. Overview of PDEs and their regulation. Circulation Research. 2007;**100**(3):309-327. DOI: 10.1161/01.RES.0000256354.95791.f1

[43] Vlachopoulos C, Terentes-Printzios D, Ioakeimidis N, et al. Beneficial effect of vardenafil on aortic stiffness and wave reflections. Journal of Clinical Pharmacology. 2012;**52**(8):1215-1221. DOI: 10.1177/0091270011413586

[44] Xu RH, Liu B, Wu JD, Yan YY, Wang JN. miR-143 is involved in endothelial cell dysfunction through suppression of glycolysis and correlated with atherosclerotic plaques formation. Eur Rev Med Pharmacol Sci. 2016;**20**(19):4063-4071

[45] Loyer X, Potteaux S, Vion AC, et al. Inhibition of microRNA-92a prevents endothelial dysfunction and atherosclerosis in mice. Circulation Research. 2014;**114**(3):434-443. DOI: 10.1161/CIRCRESAHA.114.302213

[46] Incalza MA, D'Oria R, Natalicchio A, Perrini S, Laviola L, Giorgino F. Oxidative stress and reactive oxygen species in endothelial dysfunction associated with cardiovascular and metabolic diseases. Vascular Pharmacology. 2018;**100**:1-19. DOI: 10.1016/j.vph.2017.05.005

[47] Hyndman KA, Ho DH, Sega MF, Pollock JS. Histone deacetylase 1 reduces NO production in endothelial cells via lysine deacetylation of NO synthase 3. American Journal of Physiology-Heart and Circulatory Physiology. 2014;**307**(5):H803-H809. DOI: 10.1152/ajpheart.00243.2014

[48] Balestrieri ML, Rizzo MR, Barbieri M, et al. Sirtuin 6 expression and inflammatory activity in diabetic atherosclerotic plaques: Effects of incretin treatment. Diabetes. 2015;**64**(4):1395-1406. DOI: 10.2337/db14-1149

[49] Zhang ZQ, Ren SC, Tan Y, et al. Epigenetic regulation of NKG2D ligands is involved in exacerbated atherosclerosis development in Sirt6 heterozygous mice. Scientific Reports. 2016;**6**:23912. Published 2016 Apr 5. DOI: 10.1038/srep23912

Chapter 2

An Overview of Gene Variants of Endothelin-1: A Critical Regulator of Endothelial Dysfunction

Anushree Gupta

Abstract

Endothelial dysfunction (ED) is an early marker of development of cardiovascular diseases and is closely related to clinical events in patients with atherosclerosis and hypertension. Endothelin-1 (ET-1), a potent vasoconstrictor, and nitic oxide (NO), a potent vasodilator, produced in endothelial cells are leading molecules which regulate vascular function. Failure of the physiological balance between these two molecules, often aggravated by increased production and biological activity of ET-1, commonly reflects endothelial dysfunction. The role of endothelium-derived small molecules like ET-1 (among many) with diverse biological functions continues to fascinate researchers all over the world both for its evolutionary significance and its translational potential in disease biology. Studies on systems genetics in human endothelial cells have provided evidence supporting the possibility that predisposition to complex disease is manifested through noncoding common genetic variants that modify levels of target gene expression in endothelial cells. These studies highlight the importance genetic variants of regulatory molecules secreted by endothelial cells in health and disease. It is unlikely that a single-nucleotide polymorphism (SNP) would directly cause disease, but it would increase the genetic predisposition of individuals and can affect their responses to drugs and medications. The knowledge gained would help in the risk stratification and clinical management of patients with personalized medicine.

Keywords: endothelial dysfunction, endothelin-1, cardiovascular diseases, single nucleotide polymorphisms, haplotype, precision medicine

1. Introduction

Endothelial dysfunction (ED) is a hallmark of many human vascular diseases [1] like peripheral arterial disease, cardiovascular diseases including atherosclerosis and hypertension, stroke, diabetes, chronic kidney failure, tumor growth, and metastasis. Endothelial dysfunction, like many other multifactorial diseases, is caused by a combination of multiple genetic and environmental factors, a large proportion of which remain unexplained. Individual differences in endothelial function and hence susceptibility to diseases might relate not only to different levels of exposure to risk factors but also to differences in the presence of different risk alleles of genes expressed in vascular endothelium, in different individuals [2]. Genetic regulation of variation in vascular function in different individuals is poorly understood and is largely mystifying. The genetic factors are one of the key determinants in the approach to prevent or treat diseases as envisaged by the Precision Medicine Initiative (PMI) [3] launched in 2015. Single-nucleotide polymorphisms (SNPs) are the most common genetic variation between human beings and key enablers of the concept of personalized medicine. An SNP is a single base substitution occurring at a specific site in the DNA sequence and in at least 1% or more of the population.

The healthy endothelium acts a gatekeeper of cardiovascular health regulating an exchange of fluids, nutrients, and metabolites critical to homeostasis and vascular health. Endothelial dysfunction leads to (i) loss of vascular integrity, (ii) increased expression of adhesion molecules, (iii) pro-thrombotic phenotype, (iv) production of cytokines, and (v) upregulation of human leukocyte antigen molecules [4].

Endothelial cells modulate the underlying vascular smooth muscle compartment by secreting several vasoactive substances [5] that control vascular relaxation and contraction as well as enzymes that control blood clotting, immune function, and platelet adhesion. Two major endothelium-derived factors are nitric oxide (NO) and endothelin-1 (ET-1) that have opposing effects on the function and structure of the vessel wall. Nitric oxide (NO) is a vasodilator, and endothelin (EDN-1) is a potent vasoconstrictor. Both molecules are critical regulators of vascular function. Decrease in NO production and the consequent impaired vasodilation is a hallmark of endothelial dysfunction. Failure of the complex balance between vasodilation brought about by NO and vasoconstriction brought about by ET- 1, because of genetic or acquired disturbances between these two molecules, results in changes in vascular tone and ED, triggering the pathological process of vascular diseases at their primary stage [6].

2. Genetic variation in the study of human disease

The potential of genetic discoveries in unraveling pathophysiological mechanisms and identifying drug targets is widely accepted [7]. The sequence of any two individuals is 99.5% identical, and the genomes of any two individuals differ by approximately 0.1% or less. It is in this tiny fraction of the genome that researchers seek to find the collection of sequence variations that determine susceptibility to disease and its outcome. A resource for cataloging the differences between any two genomes was created with the completion of mapping and sequencing of human genome. Sites in the DNA sequence where individuals differ at a single DNA base are called single-nucleotide polymorphisms (SNPs). As some SNPs predispose individuals to have a certain disease or trait or react to a drug in a different way, they are highly useful in diagnostics and drug development. Single-nucleotide polymorphisms (SNPs) have the potential to improve personalized medicine, and discovery of new SNPS enhance the risk stratification of patients with multifactorial diseases. In a clinical setting, SNP testing is particularly useful in complementing family history and phenotypic risk factors. The basic assumption here is that the affected individuals harbor a significant excess of clinically defined established pathogenic DNA variants as compared with a group of unaffected persons (controls) that are available from large datasets obtained from the general population.

The association of an SNP with a disease in an individual can be studied either directly or indirectly. Searching the entire genome for SNPs for disease association would be very expensive because it would involve the cost of sequencing the entire genome of several healthy and diseased individuals and comparing the sequences to identify the variants. In the indirect approach, marker SNPs called the "tag SNPs" which represent sets of nearby SNPs on the same chromosome inherited in blocks, and their disease associations are identified. The pattern of SNPs on a block is a haplotype, and a few SNPs are enough to uniquely identify the haplotypes in a block. The HapMap is a map of these haplotype blocks, and the tag SNPs are the specific SNPs that identify the haplotypes. The HapMap reduces the number of SNPs to be scanned in the genome making the indirect approach more efficient and comprehensive.

Using just the tag SNPs, particular regions of chromosomes can be identified that have different haplotype distributions in the two groups of people, those with a disease and those without. The identified regions are scanned in more detail to discover the gene variants in the region that contribute to the disease or determine the response to drugs by affecting drug metabolism pathways, leading to development of more effective tests and interventions.

The 1000 Genomes project was undertaken to provide a comprehensive description of common genetic variation by applying whole-genome sequencing to a diverse set of individuals from multiple populations. In this project, genomes of 2504 individuals from 26 populations were reconstructed by sequencing and 88 million SNPs were genotyped. The resource generated provides insights into processes that shape genetic diversity and advanced understanding of disease biology (The 1000 Genomes project Consortium, Nature 2015 [8]).

3. Candidate gene variations in endothelial dysfunction

A candidate gene in context of gene polymorphisms is one which is presumed to be associated with a particular disease or a phenotypic trait and whose biological functions are derived directly or indirectly from other studies. The role of nitric oxide (NO) and ET-1 in maintaining endothelial homeostasis is well established, and they are the obvious candidate genes of choice for studying endothelial dysfunction. Low levels of NO are associated with impaired endothelial function, and polymorphisms in genes of molecules, factors, and pathways regulating synthesis of nitric oxide in vascular endothelium have been implicated in endothelial dysfunction, the rationale being the impaired bioavailability of endogenous nitric oxide (NO) that underlies vascular disease [2]. They include polymorphisms in the endothelial nitric oxide synthase gene (eNOS gene), NOS3, asymmetric dimethyl arginine gene (*ADMA*), tetrahydrobiopterin gene *BH4*, and the gene encoding the p22phox subunit of NADPH oxidase *(CYB A)*. NO in vascular endothelium is synthesized by the enzyme NOS which requires BH4 as a co-factor. NOS is inhibited by ADMA, a naturally occurring product of metabolism found in human circulation and an analog of L-arginine. NO synthesis is inhibited by raised levels of ADMA, and this results in impaired endothelial function. Increased levels of ADMA are found in people with hypercholesterolemia, atherosclerosis, hypertension, chronic heart failure, diabetes mellitus, and chronic renal failure. Reactive oxygen species (ROS) such as superoxide (O_2^-) lead to increased inactivation of NO with the generation of $ONOO^-$ which can lead to protein and DNA damage and subsequently loss of atheroprotective functions of NO. A variant of p22phox subunit of NADPH oxidase, an enzyme responsible for generation of O_2^- in vasculature involved in the production of ROS in vessel wall, has been shown to be associated with progression of atherosclerosis [9]. Results of polymorphisms studied in other genes whose products have been implicated in endothelial dysfunction have been inconclusive.

4. Endothelin-1 as a candidate gene in human diseases for the study of endothelial dysfunction

Endothelin-1 like nitric oxide is a key regulator of endothelial dysfunction. The beneficial effects in maintenance of healthy endothelium are attributed to increased bioavailability of NO that regulates vascular homeostasis by causing vasodilation and by having antiproliferative, antioxidant, anti-inflammatory properties that inhibit atherogenesis. Conversely, increased synthesis of ET-1 is associated with the disturbance of homeostatic balance with pathological outcomes. The involvement of ET-1 in pathological process of vascular diseases with endothelial dysfunction like hypertension, coronary artery diseases, atherosclerosis, and diabetes is well established now. A knowledge of the mechanisms behind the development of endothelial dysfunction and the role of ET-1 and its gene is of great importance. The selection of ET-1 as a candidate gene is attractive because of its established role in vascular diseases and has assumed importance in the conduct of genetic association studies and SNP profiling in suitable population-based studies [10].

5. Endothelin system

The endothelin system is comprised of:

1. Endothelins (ETs): The 21 amino acid peptide isoforms such as ET-1, ET-2, and ET-3

2. Endothelin receptors (ETRs): The G-protein-coupled receptors for the peptides such as endothelin receptor A (ETRA) and endothelin receptor B (ETRB)

3. The endothelin-converting enzymes (ECEs) such as ECE1 and ECE2

5.1 Endothelin-1

Endothelin-1 was discovered as a potent vasoactive peptide [11] mainly secreted by endothelial cells and playing a role in regulating vascular tone, blood pressure, cell proliferation, and hormone production. It is now known to have diverse biological actions on almost all aspects of physiology and cell function and is increasingly being recognized as a pro-inflammatory cytokine. Because of its vasoconstricting effects on vascular smooth muscle cells (VSMCs) and the resultant increase in arterial blood pressure, the peptide is best known for its role in hypertension. It is a molecule with great clinical relevance with critical roles in neurological function [12], pulmonary physiology [13], chronic kidney disease [14], fluid and electrolyte transport [15], autoimmune disorders [16], cancer biology [17], inflammatory response and sepsis [18], embryogenesis [19, 20], and importantly endothelial dysfunction [21].

5.2 Biosynthesis of endothelin-1

ET-1 peptide is most abundant and widely expressed of the three isoforms such as ET-1, ET-2, and ET-3 [22]. ET-2 and ET-3 exhibit two and six different amino acids, respectively, compared to ET-1. ET-1 has a molecular weight of 2492, a hydrophobic carboxyl terminus, and two intramolecular disulfide bonds near the amino terminus [22]. It is the only isoform thought to be constitutively released from endothelial cells and is synthesized as the result of a series of proteolytic cleavages of the initial gene product – the preproendothelin – an inactive precursor 212 amino acids long. A 17-aa leader sequence targets preproET-1 to the endoplasmic reticulum where it enters the secretory pathway [23]. The precursor peptide is processed by furin-like proteases to biologically inert intermediates pro-endothelin1 and the 38-aa "big ET-1." Endothelin-converting enzyme (ECE) cleaves the bond between Trp^{21} and Val^{22} [24–26] to generate the mature 21-aa active ET-1 peptide (**Figure 1**).

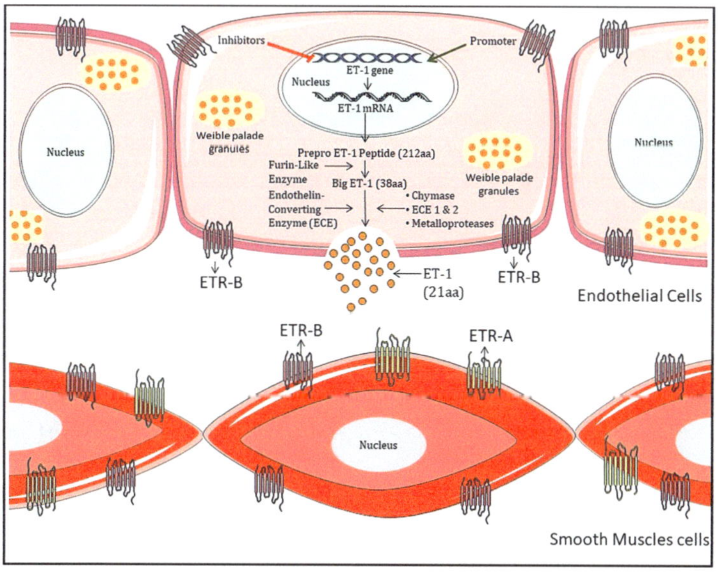

Figure 1.
Schematic representation of endothelin-1 and its biosynthesis and the localization of endothelin receptor subtypes on vascular smooth muscle cells and endothelial cells. Abbreviations: ET-1, endothelin-1; ETR-A, endothelin receptor A; ETR-B, endothelin receptor B; ECE, endothelin-converting enzyme. Figure created by using the Bioservier Medical Art.

ET-1 is synthesized by a dual pathway being released continuously by the secretory vesicles of the constitutive pathway to maintain the vascular tone [27]. They are also stored in Weibel-Palade granules of endothelial cells and released by exocytosis and degranulation in a regulated manner when exposed to pathophysiological stimuli [28].

Under physiological conditions, blood flow appears to regulate ET-1 synthesis and release via the "shear stress receptors" on endothelial cells. This endothelin synthesis is activated in response to major cardiovascular risk factors such as hyperglycemia [29, 30], hypercholesterolemia [31], arterial hypertension, estrogen deficiency [32], and aging [25], as well as by biochemical and mechanical stimuli.

5.3 Endothelin-converting enzymes

Endothelin-converting enzymes (ECE-1 and ECE-2) are type II membrane-bound zinc metalloproteases that cleave the low-activity precursor, Big ET-1 between Trp21- and Val22 to produce mature ET-1 [33]. The two enzymes have 59% overall homology [24–26, 34–36] but differ in pH for maximal activity. ECE-1 has a pH optimum of 7.0, whereas ECE-2 has an optimum pH of 5.5 for its activity. ECE-2 is 250 times more sensitive to the metalloprotease inhibitor phosphoramidon. In humans, ECE-1 has four isoforms, ECE1a-d [34, 37], derived from a single gene by differential splicing of mRNA transcripts. These isoforms differ only in the aminoacid sequence of N-terminus and show comparable efficiency in catalyzing the cleavage of Big ET-1 into mature ET-1. ECE-1 is the main enzyme responsible for the transformation of big ETs into ETs [38].

5.4 Endothelin receptors

In the vasculature, contraction or vasodilation by ET-1 are mediated by two different receptor subtypes, ET_A and ET_B [39], belonging to the family of heptahelical G-protein-coupled receptors located on vascular smooth muscle cells (VSMCs) and endothelial cells. The endothelin receptor subtypes are distinctively localized. The ETA-receptor subtype mainly mediates the vasoconstrictor activity. The receptor subtype is widely co-localized with ETR-B in vascular smooth muscle of cardiovascular tissues [40, 41], cardiopulmonary [42], central nervous system [43], retina [44], and placenta. However, ETR-A is not expressed on endothelial cells and renal-collecting duct cells. ETRB is highly expressed in the endothelium, and under pathophysiological conditions, the expression of ETB receptor subtype also increases on VSMCs and produces vasoconstriction. ETR-A has high affinity for both ET-1 and ET-2, whereas ETR-B has a similar affinity for all ET isoforms [45]. ETRB has broader effects compared to ETR-A and has roles to play in ET-1 clearance, endothelial cell survival, signaling to NO synthase (eNOS) and NO production, prostacyclin synthesis, and inhibition of ECE-1 [46]. Interaction of ET-1 with its receptors increases intracellular calcium, leading to phosphorylation and activation of myosin light chain to produce vasoconstriction [47]. Vasodilatory effect by ET-1 is mediated through ETB receptors on endothelial cells which increase the production of NO and PGI2.

Endothelin receptor antagonists (ERAs) have been developed to block the effects of ET-1 in a variety of cardiovascular conditions. Three main kinds of ERAs exist:

1. selective ETA receptor antagonists (sitaxentan, ambrisentan, atrasentan, BQ-123, and zibotentan), which affect endothelin A receptors.

2. dual antagonists (bosentan, macitentan, and tezosentan), which affect both endothelin A and B receptors.

3. selective ETB receptor antagonists (BQ-788 and A192621) which affect endothelin B receptors are used in research but have not yet reached the clinical trial stage.

Sitaxentan (withdrawn in 2010 after acute liver failure leading to death), ambrisentan, and bosentan are mainly used for the treatment of pulmonary arterial hypertension (PAH), while atrasentan is an experimental anticancer drug.

6. Possible role of endothelin in endothelial dysfunction

It is generally accepted that generation of reactive oxygen species (ROS) and an increased level of oxidative low-density lipoprotein (oxLDL) induces endothelial dysfunction. The receptor for oxidative low-density lipoprotein (oxLDL) is the lectin-like oxidized LDL receptor (LOX-1) found on endothelial cells (**Figure 2**). Under normal conditions, LOX-1 is expressed at a low level on endothelial cells, but it is induced by pro-inflammatory cytokines and under proatherogenic conditions such as hypertension, diabetes, and hyperlipidemia [6]. Angiotensin II and homocysteine that induce oxidative stress also induce LOX-1 expression. Also, LDL is oxidized by oxidative stress, leading to generation of ox-LDL. Binding of oxLDL to its receptor LOX-1 reduces NO production from endothelial cells via generation of reactive oxygen. It also induces the production of superoxide anion and activation of redox-sensitive transcription factor NFkB [48], which in turn upregulates ET-1 as well as adhesive molecules and chemokines promoting endothelial dysfunction.

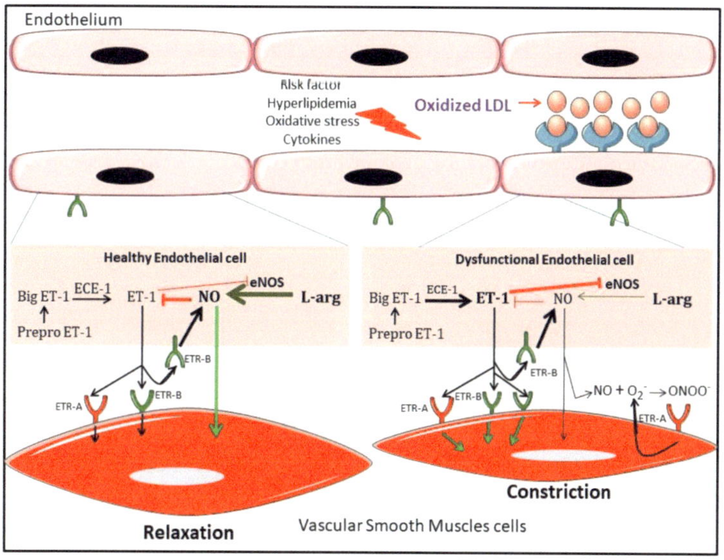

Figure 2.
The role of endothelin in endothelial dysfunction: In a healthy cell (left), the protective role of nitric oxide (NO) signaling pathway predominates. The formation of NO from L-arginine is catalyzed by endothelial NO synthase (eNOS). NO is released from endothelial cells and acts on smooth muscle cells to exert vasodilator and proliferative effects. In a dysfunctional endothelial cell (right), the vascular homeostasis is disrupted via the engagement of endothelial LOX-1 with oxidized LDL (OxLDL) resulting in downregulation of NO and upregulation of NFkB and the endothelin (ET)-1 signaling pathway. ET-1 is released from endothelial cells and acts on smooth muscle cells through the interaction of two types of receptors (ET-1 receptor type A [ETR-A] and ET-1 receptor type B [ETR-B]), both of which mediate vasoconstriction and proliferation. Figure created using Servier Medical Art.

7. Endothelin-1 gene polymorphism

An individual's phenotypic characteristics, including a person's propensity toward complex disorders such as heart disease and cancer at the genetic level, are determined by sequence variations that exist at defined positions within genomes. Sequence variations are tools for understanding human variation and molecular genetics and can be used for gene mapping, definition of population structure, and performance of functional studies. The human genome has a total of over 88 million variants of which 84.7 million are SNPs, 3.6 million short insertions/deletions (indels), and 60,000 structural variants (The 1000 Genomes Project Consortium, Nature, 2015 [8]). A typical genome differs from the reference human genome at 4.1million–5.0 million sites. Realizing the importance of the role of SNPs in human health, many databases like Ensembl Variation Database, A-SNP, HGBase (Human Genic Bi-allelic SEquences), HOWDY (Human organized whole-genome variation Database), and dbSNP have been created for cataloging the variations occurring in human genome. The emergence of genetic variation databases, such as (i) dbSNP and HGV for short genetic variations, (ii) dbVar and DGV for structural variations, (iii) dbGaP for genotype/phenotype interaction studies, and (iv) ClinVar and ClinGen for human variations of clinical significance, facilitates the contemporary identification/discovery of (i) known or novel polymorphisms, (ii) phenotype to genotype associations, and (iii) clinically important human genetic variations.

The Single Nucleotide Polymorphism Database (dbSNP) is **a free public archive for genetic variation** developed and hosted by the National Centre for Biotechnology Information (NCBI) in collaboration with the National Human Genome Research Institute (NHGRI). This collection of polymorphisms includes

i. single-base nucleotide substitutions (also known as single-nucleotide polymorphisms or SNPs),

ii. small-scale multi-base deletions or insertions (also called deletion insertion polymorphisms or DIPs), and

iii. retrotransposable element insertions and microsatellite repeat variations (also called short tandem repeats or STRs).

Majority of the genetic variations among individuals are due to SNPs. The association of candidate gene SNPs like those of EDN1 in multifactorial diseases, like endothelial dysfunction which often set the stage for the occurrence of vascular diseases like CAD, is important for the identification of therapeutic targets.

The gene for ET-1 gene locus spans a region of approx. 7.0 kb on short arm of chromosome 6 at 6p24–23 [49, 50]. The gene is composed of five exons (**Figure 3**) that synthesizes a cDNA of 2026 bps. Nucleotide sequences encoding the mature ET-1 are present in the second exon. ExonI has the 5'UTR of mRNA. The upstream promoter region is well conserved.

The endothelin pathway is central to pulmonary vascular function. Several polymorphisms and/or mutations in the genes coding for endothelin (ET)-1 and its receptors correlate with the clinical manifestations of other diseases. The dbSNP contains 15,259 entries for human *EDN1* gene (as on 20.06.2022) which represent

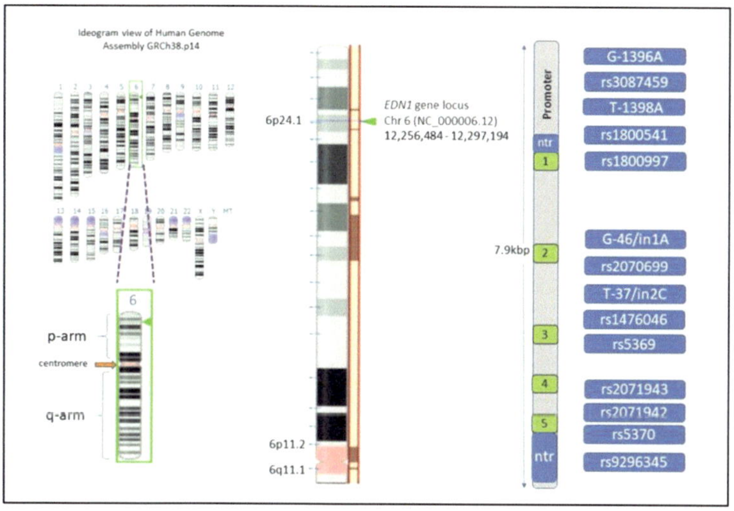

Figure 3.
EDN1 Gene Locus and some of its common gene variants. The EDN1 gene is located on short arm (p-arm) of chromosome 6 and has five exons (green), a 5'non-translated region and a 3'non-translated region of the gene that is transcribed in mRNA. The 5'ntr is located downstream of promoter, while the 3'ntr is located downstream of exon 5. The gray areas of the gene represent the introns that are spliced off in the mature RNA. The rs nos. of commonly studied SNP variants in EDN1 gene are mentioned in blue horizontal bars in extreme right. The complete data from SNPs build 155 are available at https://ftp.ncbi.nlm.nih.gov/snp/ in multiple formats.

all the above categories of variations. Many of these entries are redundant. For example, rs386556298, rs60458956, rs56478068, and rs3730357 have been merged into rs2070699 which represents intron variant c.233 + 30 G > C/G > T variation in the *EDN1* gene. A total of 15 of these as represented in the ClinVar database (Build 155, Jun 16, 2021) have been included in **Table 1** due to the limitation of space in this article.

This is by far the most reported variant of pre-proendothelin-1, and there are 161 publications (21.06.2022) in LitVar for this variant. The third base "**G**" of codon 198 of preproendothelin-1 gene is substituted with "**T**" leading to a change in codon for lysine to arginine. The genotypic variants of rs5370 are GG, GT, and TT. In the ECTIM (**Etude Cas-Témoin de l'Infarctus du Myocarde**) multicenter study [51] comprising of 648 male patients who had survived myocardial infarction and 760 population-based controls, the G/T polymorphism predicting the Lys/Asn change showed that the "T" allele was associated with increase of blood pressure in overweight subjects. This finding was confirmed by the Glasgow Heart Scan Study [51] as well.

7.1 Pulmonary arterial hypertension

Endothelial dysfunction is believed to be one of the first triggers initiating the process of abnormal vascular remodeling in pulmonary arterial hypertension (PAH) [52]. K198N (rs5370) polymorphism in the endothelin 1 gene (EDN1) has been demonstrated to associate with blood pressure reactivity and can result in greater endothelin-1 (ET-1) synthesis which may favor the development of PAH and affect its course of progression [53]. The influence of EDN1 gene variants on susceptibility to pulmonary arterial hypertension remains uncertain. However, a meta-analysis of

S.No.	Variant	Alleles	Coding/noncoding	Position	Flanks (25 nt. on either side of the SNP site)	Amino acid
1	rs376892399	G>A, T	Coding/synonymous	g.8658 c.246	5' CTTTGGATAA TAGGCACGTT GTTCC[G/A/T] 3' TATGGACTTG GAAGCCCTAG GTCCA	Pro 82=P[CCG] > P [CCA]
2	rs 10478695	C>A,G,T	Intron	g.5406	5' AAGGAGCTCC AGAAACAGGT AGGCA[C/A/G/T] 3' GCTCGTTGAC TTGTAAGTCT CGGAA	
3	rs147381256	G>A	Coding/missense	g.8650 c.238	5' CTITCTCTCT TTGGATAATA GGCAC[G/A] 3' TTGTTCCGTA TGGACTTGGA AGCOC	Val 79 lle V[GTT] > I [ATT]
4	rs145546137	A>C	Coding/missense	g.9056 c.480	5' GGAAAAAGTG TATITATCAG CAGTT[A/C] 3' GTGAGAGGAA GAAAAATCAG AAGAA	Leu 160 Phe L[TTA] > F[TTC]
5	rs183694577	G>A,C	Coding/missense	g.7087 c.106	5' GCTCAGCGCG GTGGGTGAGA ACGGC[G/A/C] 3' GGGAGAAACC CACTCCCAGT CCACC	Gly36Arg G[GGG] > R[AGG]
6	rs 150035515	G>A,T	Coding/synonymous	g.7071 c.90	5' CAGTCTTAGG CGCTGAGCTC AGCGC[G/A/T] 3' GTGGGTGAGA ACGGCGGGGA GAAAC	Ala30 = A[GCG] > [GCA]
7	rs148565651	C>T	Coding/synonymous	g.7122 c.141	5' CCACTCCCAG TCCACCCTGG CGGCT[C/T] 3' CGCCGGTCCA AGCGCTGCTC CTGCT	LEU47 = L[CTC] > L[CTT]
8	rs1561693994	G>C	Coding/missense	g.7165 c.184	5' CTCCTGCTCG TCCCTTGATGG ATAAA[G/C] 3' AGTGTGTCTA CTTCTGCCAC CTGGA	Glu62Gln E[GAG] > Q[CAG]
9	rs149316725	C>A	Coding/missense	g.9093 c.517	5' AAAAATCAGA AGAAGTTCAG AGGAA[C/A] 3' ACCTAAGACA AACCAGGTAA GAGGG	His173Asn H[CAC] > N[AAC]
10	rs1064796796	G>A	Coding/missense	g.7169 c.188	5' TGCTCGTCCC TGATGGATAA AGAGT[G/A] 3' TGTCTACTTC TGCCACCTGG ACATC	Cys63Tyr C [TGT] > Y [TAT]
11	rs587777231	A>G	Coding/missense	g.8683 C.271	5' GTATGGACTT GGAAGCCCTA GGTCC[A/G] 3' AGAGAGCCTT GGAGAATITA CTICC	Lys91Glu K [AAG] > E[GAG}
12	rs587777232	C>A	Coding/missense	g.7211 C.230	5' CTGGACATCA TITGGGTCAA CACTC[C/A] 3' CGAGTAAGIC TCTAGAGGGC ATTGT	Pro77His P[CCC] > H[CAC]
13	rs587777233	T>A	Coding/missense	g.7172 c.191	5' TCGTCCCTGA TGGATAAAGA GTGTG[T/A] 3' CTACTTCTGC CACCTGGACA TCATT	Val64Asp V[GTC] > D[GAC]

14	rs587777234	T>G	Coding/stop_gained	g.8661 c.249	5' TGGATAATAG GCACGTTGTT CCGTA[T/G] 3' GGACTTGGAA GCCCTAGGTC CAAGA	Tyr83Termination Y[T A T] > * [TAG]
15	rs5370	G>T	Coding/missense	c.594	5' TTCATGATCC CAAGCTGAAA GGCAA[G/T] 3' CCCTCCAGAG AGCGTTATGT GACCC	Lys198Asn K[AAG] > N [AAT]

rs5370: Codon 198: Lys198Asn or K198N (G > T Transversion in Exon 5 Position g.10727 of RefSeqGene NG_016196.1 and position c.594 of transcript variant 1 NM_001955.5 and position c.591 of transcript variant 2 NM_001168319.2).

Table 1.
15 SNP variants reported in Clinvar database having pathophysiological significance are mentioned with their rs I'd, allelic variation, their occurrence in coding vs. noncoding region in the gene, their coordinates, and 25 nucleotide upstream and the downstream flanking sequences and the amino acid change associated with SNPs in the exonic/coding region. SNPs mentioned here are from transcript variant 1 (NM_001955.5) and the corresponding genomic RefSeq EDN1 gene (NG_016196.1). Among 15 SNPs, 5 are benign, 3 are likely benign, 3 are of uncertain significance, and 4 are pathogenic. One of the SNP rs5370 G > T has multiple submitters. The complete data from SNPs build 155 are available at https://ftp.ncbi.nlm.nih.gov/snp/ in multiple formats.

a total of 17 articles with 2631PAH subjects and 5139 controls and 5 candidate gene variants that also included rs5370 SNP of EDN1 gene for susceptibility to PAH showed a significant association between "T" allele carriers and risk of developing PAH [54]. Another large-scale genomic analysis to examine the interaction of ET-1 pathway polymorphisms and treatment response of patients with PAH treated with ET receptor anatagonists (ERAs) showed that these polymorphisms of the ET-1 pathway may influence the clinical efficacy of ERAs [55].

7.2 Essential hypertension

There are several reports connecting this SNP variant to hypertension. Our own studies (unpublished) like those of Wiltshire et al. [43] have found no sufficient data supporting the association between K198N polymorphism with high blood pressure, systolic blood pressure, lipid levels, and insulin resistance or metabolic syndrome. In other studies, subjects with high endothelin-1 levels were shown to have an increased risk of low-renin hypertension [56]. Rs5370 variant of EDN1 has been associated with low-renin hypertension and increased aldosterone/renin ratios in individuals of African descent, but not in whites [57]. This study also provided the first evidence of a potential association between the *EDN1* rs5370 SNP and the risk of subclinical hyperaldosteronism in subjects of African descent. These investigators also assessed the effect of EDN1 rs5370 on systolic BP curves, but they did not see an effect. They also observed a significant association of salt-sensitive BP and rs5370, even with adjustment for sex, since an earlier study [58] had reported sex differences in the relationship between systolic BP and a haplotype of *EDN1.* In rheumatoid arthritis, hypertension is quite common and has been reported to be associated with the endothelin-1 (ET-1) gene locus (EDN1) in some groups, such as the Afro-Caribbean but not in the general population. Some other groups where hypertension-related high levels of plasma ET-1 in RA have been observed are the obese and individuals with low-renin states. A study [59] that evaluated the potential association of EDN1 gene locus and serum ET-1 levels with hypertension in patients with RA showed an increase in the prevalence of T-T haplotype carriers.

7.3 Preeclampsia

Preeclampsia (PE) is an often-fatal pathology characterized by hypertension and proteinuria at the 20th week of gestation that affects 5–10% of the pregnancies [46]. Risk factors for the development of PE include obesity, insulin resistance, and hyperlipidemia that stimulate inflammatory cytokine release and oxidative stress leading to endothelial dysfunction (ED). Normal pregnancy course includes variations in hemodynamics, in which placenta allows the exchange of nutrients and waste disposal between mother and fetus. During the stage of establishment of maternal-fetal interface when the extravillous throphoblasts from placenta conquer the maternal decidua, the maternal spiral arteries from the decidua go through a process of remodeling, where they are upgraded from low-capacity high-resistance into high-capacity low-resistance vessels. PE is characterized by an impaired invasion of fetal trophoblasts which causes a reduced remodeling of the maternal spiral arteries eventually leading to a decrease in blood flow to the placenta. Consequently, the mother develops hypertension, usually at the end of the second or third trimester of gestation, to increase the blood flow. The polymorphism rs5370 in EDN1 was shown to be associated with susceptibility to preeclampsia [60]. In another study [61], markedly increased risk of early onset of PE was shown to be related to the C allele polymorphism rs5370 in *EDN1.*

7.4 Glaucoma

ET-1 has been suggested to have a role to play in optic neuropathy observed in glaucoma [62]. Associations between polymorphisms of endothelin (ET-1) and endothelin receptors (ER) A and B genes with the occurrence of glaucoma were investigated by Ishikawa et al. [63] in Japanese patients. For the rs5370 ET-1 polymorphism that involved a transversion of G/T in exon 5, the Lys-Lys (GG) genotype tended to be more frequent than in open-angle glaucoma patients.

7.5 Diabetic retinopathy (DR)

Diabetic retinopathy (DR) is the result of impaired NO pathway that affects the vusculature of the retina. Several candidate genes have been studied for their role in diabetic retinopathy, but only a fraction of them have been shown to be associated with DR. Many studies have provided evidence in support of the role of endothelin (ET) system in the pathophysiology of DN. However, studies on K198N variant have revealed that the "T" (Asn) allele actually has a protective role against DR in a Chinese population with type 2 diabetes [64]. Yet another study by Maja Seruga [65] showed that the EDN1 rs5370, rs1476046, and rs3087459 polymorphisms of EDN1 gene are not risk factors for DN in Caucasians with T2DM.

7.6 Childhood primary nephrotic syndrome

ET-1 levels are raised in children with first episode of nephrotic syndrome (FENS), pointing toward endothelial dysfunction [66]. Also, children with steroid resistance have a greater risk of endothelial dysfunction [67]. The rs5730 SNP of EDN1 gene might play a disease-modifying role and susceptibility to childhood primary nephrotic syndrome (CPNS) [68]. Plasma Cholesterol, a hallmark of NS, seems to be associated with the genetic variations within the human ET-1 gene. The other EDN1 SNPs associated with CPNS include rs1630736 and rs10478694 (3A/4A) and rs9296344 [69]. In a case-control study, it was found that GG genotype was more frequent in steroid-sensitive NS group compared to the steroid-resistant NS group and was associated with hypertension. This group also showed a better response to steroid therapy [70]. The study by Hashemi et al. [71], however, did not find any association of rs5370 G > T variant with nephrotic syndrome in children.

7.7 Asthma

EDN1 has been reported to be implicated in the pathophysiology of asthma. In a study on 342 families from UK and 100 families from Norway, rs5370 along with 10 other EDN1 variants rs1800541, rs1800542, rs1476046, rs1800543, rs5369, rs1794849, rs1626492, rs1629862, rs1630736, and rs4714383 were genotyped, and a strong association was found in both the populations for rs5370 and rs1800541 located in the upstream region of EDN1 gene [72]. However, literature results on the genetic association of EDN1 in asthma are inconsistent.

7.8 As risk predictors in cancer

Ma et al. analyzed the genotypes of angiogenesis-related genes in 180 patients with nasopharyngeal carcinoma (NPC) using Sequenom MassARRAY and found that EDN1-rs1800541, rs2071942, and rs5370 can be used as risk predictors of radiation-induced oral mucositis, xerostomia, and myelosuppression, respectively.

Auriculocondylar Syndrome and Question Mark Ears.

rs587777231 [Lys91Glu].

rs587777232[Pro71His].

rs587777233[Val64Asp],

rs587777234 [Tyr81 Termination (stop gained)].

Auriculocondylar syndrome (ACS) is a rare disorder which affects facial development with a small chin micro-gnatha) and a malfunction of the joint that connects the lower jaw (mandible) to the skull—a condition referred to as mandibular hypoplasia. Another feature of this disorder is malformed outer ears that have a characteristic shape caused by a split that separates the upper ear from the earlobe (question-mark ears or QMEs). Ref. [73] identified a homozygous substitution in a furin cleavage site of the EDN1 proprotein in ACS-affected siblings born to consanguineous parents by whole-exome sequencing (WES). Four mutations (S.No. 11–14 in the ClinVar Table) were identified in the EDN1 gene, one of which resulted in a stop codon and the other three resulted in missense mutations. These mutations also had different modes of inheritance, suggesting that the degree of residual EDN1 activity differed depending on the mutation. These findings provided support for the hypothesis that ACS and QMEs are uniquely caused by disruption of the EDN1-EDNRA signaling pathway which is important in the development of the lower jaw. The four variants are classified in ClinVar database as pathogenic having clinical manifestations.

rs1800997: 3A/4A (+138 5'UTR locus of exon1 ins/del A) polymorphism.

(Formerly rs10478694)

This SNP contains an adenine insertion at position +138, 5′ untranslated region (UTR) and exon 1 of the ET-1 [74]. The genotypes are as follows: the mutant form (4A/4A), wild type (3A/3A), and the heterozygote (3A/4A) [53]. Some studies have reported increased plasma levels of ET-1 in individuals who have a mutant genotype [53, 75]. Studies have reported different allele distributions among patients with pulmonary artery hypertension (PAH), idiopathic pulmonary artery hypertension (IPAH), and coronary heart disease (CHD), with the control group [76]. They showed a significant increase of alleles containing the 3A form in patients with hypertension [76]. Some researchers have shown that there is no significant association between this SNP and the development of hypertension [77]. This SNP, although, not reported in ClinVar database has been shown to be associated with high expression levels of ET-1 both in vitro (Popowski) and in vivo (Abhishek Kumar, 2021), and the high expression levels associated with the homozygous mutant form 4A/4A were hypothesized to be deleterious to cyanotic children with severe pulmonary hypertension [75].

Other variants not reported in ClinVar Database but reported in literature as heritable risk variants in many cardiovascular disorders such as hypertension, coronary artery disease, ventricular arrhythmia, and other related disorders are shown in **Figure 3**.

8. Summary and conclusions

Endothelial dysfunction is multifactorial, and ET-1 is a key regulator of ED. The genetic factors that modulate individual susceptibility to multifactorial diseases are common, functionally different forms of genes (polymorphisms), that have modest effects on physiology and disease biology at individual level but, because of their high frequency of occurrence in the population, can be associated with a high attributable risk. By definition, a mutation results in a significant phenotype, whereas an SNP, which represents a stable change in the genome, possesses mild or no phenotypic changes. SNPs whether they relate clinical end points or intermediate phenotypes such as endothelial dysfunction require careful analysis. Available evidence in literature suggests that most of the susceptibility genes from common diseases do not have a primary etilogical role in predisposition to disease, but rather act as response modifiers to exogenous factors such as stress, environment, disease, and drug intake. A better characterization of the interactions between environmental and genetic factors constitute a key issue in understanding of the pathogenesis of multifactorial diseases. For example, risk factors like oxidative stress, hyperlipidemia, and cytokines disrupt the vascular homeostasis in a dysfunctional endothelial cell leading to the production of ET-1 and consequent pathophysiological changes. Also, results from two independent studies ECTIM and Glasgow Heart Scan Study [53] on ET-1, BMI, and Blood Pressure suggested that obesity is a crucial factor influencing the association between the ET-1/ Lys198Asn polymorphism and BP levels. Obesity, predominantly governed by complex social and environmental factors, might enhance expression of ET-1 gene possibly through an upregulation by insulin, which is known to stimulate ET-1 production [78]. In common diseases, genetic effects can be considerably amplified in the presence of triggering factors and gene-environment interaction is a central concept in multifactorial diseases.

The potential usefulness of SNPs in medicine is unprecedented. Obtaining a detailed family history is often considered standard in clinical practice for characterizing the inherited component of individual's disease risk. SNPs allow us to look closely at the footprints of past generations of the families. SNPs of the endothelin-1 gene axis have the potential to help us in dissecting the genetic component of complex diseases like cardiovascular diseases of which vascular dysfunction is an early manifestation. Susceptibility to disease in such cases depends on the cumulative contribution of multiple genetic risk factors. SNPs provide the potential to interpret genetic risks associated with complex polygenic disorders by developing models based on quantitative genetic theory to analyze and compare family history and SNP-based models [79, 80].

The most difficult task will be to consider the implementation of SNPs in clinical decision-making, particularly as it relates to providing recommendations for interventional or preventional measures, based on the concept of "risk."

Acknowledgements

The author appreciates and thanks Mr. Shubham kumar Agrawal and Mr. Bhaskar Saxena, M.Biotech. students of batches 2021 and 2022, respectively, of Department of Biotechnology, AIIMS, New Delhi, for their efforts in preparation and layout of figures and compilation of references for the chapter.

List of abbreviations

ET-1	Endothelin-1
ETRA	Endothelin Receptor A
ETRB	Endothelin Receptor B
ECEs	Endothelin-Converting Enzymes
ERAs	Endothelin Receptor Antagonists
NO	Nitric Oxide
eNOS	Endothelial NO Synthase
OxLDL	Oxidized LDL
SPH	Severe Pulmonary Hypertension,
CHD	Congenital Heart Disease
SNPs	Single Nucleotide Polymorphisms,
5'UTR	5'Untranslated Region
In/del	Insertion/Deletion
WES	Whole-Exome Sequencing
PE	Preeclampsia
DR	Diabetic Retinopathy
FENS	First Episode Of Nephrotic Syndrome
CPNS	Childhood Primary Nephrotic Syndrome
ACS	Auriculocondylar syndrome
QMEs	Question-Mark Ears

Author details

Anushree Gupta
Biotechnology, All India Institute of Medical Sciences, New Delhi, India

*Address all correspondence to: anushree.gupta@gmail.com

IntechOpen

© 2022 The Author(s). Licensee IntechOpen. This chapter is distributed under the terms of the Creative Commons Attribution License (http://creativecommons.org/licenses/by/3.0), which permits unrestricted use, distribution, and reproduction in any medium, provided the original work is properly cited.

References

[1] Cahill PA, Redmond EM. Vascular endothelium - Gatekeeper of vessel health. Atherosclerosis. 2016;**248**:97-109

[2] Jones LC, Hingorani AD. Genetic regulation of endothelial function. Heart. 2005;**91**(10):1275-1277

[3] Collins FS, Varmus H. A new initiative on precision medicine. NEJM. 2015;**372**(9):793-795

[4] Hunt BJ, Jurd KM. Endothelial cell activation. A central pathophysiological process. BMJ. 1998;**316**(7141):1328-1329

[5] Hickey KA et al. Characterization of a coronary vasoconstrictor produced by cultured endothelial cells. The American Journal of Physiology. 1985;**248**(5 Pt 1): C550-C556

[6] Sakurai K, Sawamura T. Stress and vascular responses: Endothelial dysfunction via lectin-like oxidized low-density lipoprotein receptor-1: Close relationships with oxidative stress. Journal of Pharmacological Sciences. 2003;**91**(3):182-186

[7] Nelson MR et al. The support of human genetic evidence for approved drug indications. Nature Genetics. 2015;**47**(8):856-860

[8] Genomes Project C et al. A global reference for human genetic variation. Nature. 2015;**526**(7571):68-74

[9] Cahilly C et al. A variant of p22(phox), involved in generation of reactive oxygen species in the vessel wall, is associated with progression of coronary atherosclerosis. Circulation Research. 2000;**86**(4):391-395

[10] Abraham G, Inouye M. Genomic risk prediction of complex human disease and its clinical application. Current Opinion in Genetics & Development. 2015;**33**:10-16

[11] Yanagisawa M, Kurihara H, Kimura S, Tomobe Y, Kobayashi M, Mitsui Y, et al. A novel potent vasoconstrictor peptide produced by vascular endothelial cells. Nature 1988;**332**(6163):411-415

[12] Dashwood MR, Loesch A. Endothelin-1 as a neuropeptide: Neurotransmitter or neurovascular effects? Journal of Cell Communication and Signaling. 2010;**4**(1):51-62

[13] Abman SH. Pulmonary hypertension in children: A historical overview. Pediatric Critical Care Medicine. 2010;**11**(2 Suppl):S4-S9

[14] Barton M. Reversal of proteinuric renal disease and the emerging role of endothelin. Nature Clinical Practice. Nephrology. 2008;**4**(9):490-501

[15] Kohan DE. Biology of endothelin receptors in the collecting duct. Kidney International. 2009;**76**(5):481-486

[16] Neuhofer, W. and D. Pittrow, Endothelin in human autoimmune diseases with renal involvement. Rheumatology (Oxford), 2006;**45**(Suppl 3):iii39-iii41

[17] Rosano L, Spinella F, Bagnato A. Endothelin 1 in cancer: Biological implications and therapeutic opportunities. Nature Reviews. Cancer. 2013;**13**(9):637-651

[18] Kowalczyk A et al. The role of endothelin-1 and endothelin receptor antagonists in inflammatory response and sepsis. Archivum Immunologiae

et Therapiae Experimentalis (Warsz). 2015;**63**(1):41-52

[19] Bonano M et al. A new role for the Endothelin-1/Endothelin-A receptor signaling during early neural crest specification. Developmental Biology. 2008;**323**(1):114-129

[20] Mihanfar A et al. Endothelins and their receptors in embryo implantation. Journal of Cellular Biochemistry. 2019:1-11

[21] Masaki T, Sawamura T. Endothelin and endothelial dysfunction. Proceedings of the Japan Academy. Series B, Physical and Biological Sciences. 2006;**82**(1):17-24

[22] Yanagisawa M, Masaki T. Molecular biology and biochemistry of the endothelins. Trends in Pharmacological Sciences. 1989;**10**(9):374-378

[23] Fabbrini MS et al. The signal peptide of human preproendothelin-1. FEBS Letters. 1991;**286**(1-2):91-94

[24] Shimada K, Matsushita Y, Wakabayashi K, Takahashi M, Matsubara A, Iijima Y, et al. Cloning and functional expression of human endothelin-converting enzyme cDNA. Biochemical and Biophysical Research Communications. 1995b;**207**:807-812

[25] Stauffer BL, Westby CM, DeSouza CA. Endothelin-1, aging and hypertension. Current Opinion in Cardiology. 2008;**23**(4):350-355

[26] Emoto N, Yanagisawa M. Endothelin-converting enzyme-2 is a membrane-bound, phosphoramidon-sensitive metalloprotease with acidic pH optimum. The Journal of Biological Chemistry. 1995;**270**(25):15262-15268

[27] Haynes WG, Webb DJ. Contribution of endogenous generation of endothelin-1 to basal vascular tone. Lancet. 1994;**344**(8926):852-854

[28] Russell FD, Coppell AL, Davenport AP. In vitro enzymatic processing of radiolabelled big ET-1 in human kidney. Biochemical Pharmacology. 1998;**55**(5):697-701

[29] Manea SA, Todirita A, Manea A. High glucose-induced increased expression of endothelin-1 in human endothelial cells is mediated by activated CCAAT/enhancer-binding proteins. PLoS One. 2013;**8**(12):e84170

[30] Cardillo UC, Bryant MB, Julio A. Panza increased activity of endogenous endothelin in patients with Type II diabetes mellitus carmine. Circulation. 2002;**106**:1783-1787

[31] Cardillo C et al. Increased activity of endogenous endothelin in patients with hypercholesterolemia. Journal of the American College of Cardiology. 2000;**36**(5):1483-1488

[32] Akishita M et al. Estrogen inhibits endothelin-1 production and c-fos gene expression in rat aorta. Atherosclerosis. 1996;**125**(1):27

[33] Xu D, Emoto N, Giaid A, Slaughter C, Kaw S, deWit D, et al. ECE-1: A membrane-bound metalloprotease that catalyzes the proteolytic activation of big endothelin-1. Cell. 1994;**78**(3):473-485

[34] Schweizer A et al. Human endothelin-converting enzyme (ECE-1): Three isoforms with distinct subcellular localizations. The Biochemical Journal. 1997;**328**(Pt 3):871-877

[35] Vargas-Alarcon G et al. The -974C>A (rs3087459) gene polymorphism in the endothelin gene (EDN1) is associated with risk of developing acute coronary

syndrome in Mexican patients. Gene. 2014;**542**(2):258-262

[36] Yorimitsu K, Moroi K, Inagaki N, Saito T, Masuda Y, Masaki T, et al. Cloning and sequencing of a human endothelin-converting enzyme in renal adenocarcinoma (ACHN) cells producing endothelin-2. Biochemical and Biophysical Research Communications. 1995;**208**:721-727

[37] Valdenaire O et al. A fourth isoform of endothelin-converting enzyme (ECE-1) is generated from an additional promoter molecular cloning and characterization. European Journal of Biochemistry. 1999;**264**(2):341-349

[38] Yanagisawa H, Yanagisawa M, Kapur RP, Richardson JA, Williams SC, Clouthier DE, et al. Dual genetic pathways of endothelin-mediated intercellular signaling revealed by targeted disruption of endothelin converting enzyme-1 gene. Development. 1998;**125**:825-836

[39] Davenport AP, Battistini B. Classification of endothelin receptors and antagonists in clinical development. Clinical Science (London, England). 2002;**103**(Suppl. 48):1S-3S

[40] Adachi M et al. Cloning and characterization of cDNA encoding human A-type endothelin receptor. Biochemical and Biophysical Research Communications. 1991;**180**(3):1265-1272

[41] Hosoda K et al. Cloning and expression of human endothelin-1 receptor cDNA. FEBS Letters. 1991;**287**(1-2):23-26

[42] Hemsen A et al. Occurrence, specific binding sites and functional effects of endothelin in human cardiopulmonary tissue. European Journal of Pharmacology. 1990;**191**(3):319-328

[43] Wiltshire S et al. Investigating the association between K198N coding polymorphism in EDN1 and hypertension, lipoprotein levels, the metabolic syndrome and cardiovascular disease. Human Genetics. 2008;**123**(3):307-313

[44] MacCumber MW, D'Anna SA. Endothelin receptor-binding subtypes in the human retina and choroid. Archives of Ophthalmology. 1994;**112**(9):1231-1235

[45] Khimji AK, Rockey DC. Endothelin--biology and disease. Cellular Signalling. 2010;**22**(11):1615-1625

[46] Sanchez-Aranguren LC et al. Endothelial dysfunction and preeclampsia: Role of oxidative stress. Frontiers in Physiology. 2014;**5**:372

[47] Pollock DM, Keith TL, Highsmith RF. Endothelin receptors and calcium signaling. The FASEB Journal. 1995;**9**(12):1196-1204

[48] Cominacini L et al. Oxidized low density lipoprotein (ox-LDL) binding to ox-LDL receptor-1 in endothelial cells induces the activation of NF-kappaB through an increased production of intracellular reactive oxygen species. The Journal of Biological Chemistry. 2000;**275**(17):12633-12638

[49] Bloch KD et al. cDNA cloning and chromosomal assignment of the gene encoding endothelin 3. The Journal of Biological Chemistry. 1989;**264**(30):18156-18161

[50] Arinami T et al. Chromosomal assignments of the human endothelin family genes: the endothelin-1 gene (EDN1) to 6p23-p24, the endothelin-2 gene (EDN2) to 1p34, and the endothelin-3 gene (EDN3) to

20q13.2-q13.3. American Journal of Human Genetics. 1991;**48**(5):990-996

[51] Tiret L et al. The Lys198Asn polymorphism in the endothelin-1 gene is associated with blood pressure in overweight people. Hypertension. 1999;**33**(5):1169-1174

[52] Kurakula K et al. Endothelial dysfunction in pulmonary hypertension: Cause or consequence? Biomedicine. 2021;**9**(1):1-23

[53] Vadapalli S et al. Endothelin-1 and endothelial nitric oxide polymorphisms in idiopathic pulmonary arterial hypertension. International Journal of Molecular Epidemiology and Genetics. 2010;**1**(3):208-213

[54] Jiao YR et al. 5-HTT, BMPR2, EDN1, ENG, KCNA5 gene polymorphisms and susceptibility to pulmonary arterial hypertension: A meta-analysis. Gene. 2019;**680**:34-42

[55] Benza RL et al. Endothelin-1 pathway polymorphisms and outcomes in pulmonary arterial hypertension. American Journal of Respiratory and Critical Care Medicine. 2015;**192**(11):1345-1354

[56] Letizia C et al. High plasma endothelin-1 levels in hypertensive patients with low-renin essential hypertension. Journal of Human Hypertension. 1997;**11**(7):447-451

[57] Tan JW et al. Dysregulated aldosterone secretion in persons of African descent with endothelin-1 gene variants. JCI Insight. 2017;**2**(23):1-12

[58] Dong Y et al. Endothelin-1 gene and progression of blood pressure and left ventricular mass: Longitudinal findings in youth. Hypertension. 2004;**44**(6):884-890

[59] Panoulas VF et al. Polymorphisms of the endothelin-1 gene associate with hypertension in patients with rheumatoid arthritis. Endothelium. 2008;**15**(4):203-212

[60] Seremak-Mrozikiewicz A et al. Genetic variability of endothelin-1 system in gestational hypertension and preeclampsia. Ginekologia Polska. 2011;**82**(5):363-370

[61] Li J, Yin W, Liu M-S, Mao L-J, Wang X-H. Potential correlation between EDN1 gene polymorphisms with preeclampsia. European Review for Medical and Pharmacological Sciences. 2020;**24**(4):1602-1608

[62] Yorio T, Krishnamoorthy R, Prasanna G. Endothelin: Is it a contributor to glaucoma pathophysiology? Journal of Glaucoma. 2002;**11**(3):259-270

[63] Ishikawa K, Funayama T, Ohtake Y, Kimura I, Ideta H, Nakamoto K, et al. Association between glaucoma and gene polymorphism of endothelin type a receptor. Molecular Vision. 2005;**11**:431-437

[64] Li H et al. EDN1 Lys198Asn is associated with diabetic retinopathy in type 2 diabetes. Molecular Vision. 2008;**14**:1698-1704

[65] Seruga M et al. Endothelin-1 gene polymorphisms rs5370, rs1476046, and rs3087459 are not associated with diabetic nephropathy in caucasians with type 2 diabetes mellitus. Folia Medica (Plovdiv). 2017;**59**(3):261-269

[66] Arumugam V, Saha A, Kaur M, Kapoor K, Arora N, Basak T, et al. Ashish Datt Upadhyay, Endothelin 1 and endothelial dysfunction in children with idiopathic nephrotic syndrome. Artery Research. 2017;**18**:36-40

[67] Bhatia A, Saha A, Deepthi B, Goyal P, Upadhyay AD, Dubey NK. Endothelial dysfunction in children with frequently relapsing and steroid-resistant nephrotic syndrome. Asian Journal of Paediatric Nephrology. 2020;**3**:4-9

[68] Yang F, Lai X, Deng L, et al. Association of endothelin-1 gene polymorphisms with the clinical phenotype in primary nephrotic syndrome of children. Life Sciences. 2014;**118**(2):446-450

[69] Zhang R et al. Endothelin-1 rs9296344 associates with the susceptibility of childhood primary nephrotic syndrome. Journal of Clinical Laboratory Analysis. 2020;**34**(4): e23134

[70] Rizk H et al. Endothelin-1 rs5370 gene polymorphism in primary nephrotic syndrome: A case-control study. Anales de Pediatría (English Edition). 2020

[71] Hashemi M et al. Association of Endothelin-1 rs5370 G>T gene polymorphism with the risk of nephrotic syndrome in children. Journal of Nephropathology. 2017;**6**(3):138-143

[72] Zhu G et al. Polymorphisms in the endothelin-1 (EDN1) are associated with asthma in two populations. Genes and Immunity. 2008;**9**(1):23-29

[73] Gordon CT et al. Heterogeneity of mutational mechanisms and modes of inheritance in auriculocondylar syndrome. Journal of Medical Genetics. 2013;**50**(3):174-186

[74] Diefenbach K et al. Identification of twelve polymorphisms in the endothelin-1 gene by use of fluorescently labeled oligonucleotides and PCR with restriction fragment polymorphism analysis. Clinical Chemistry. 2004;**50**(2):448-451

[75] Kumar A et al. In vivo assessment of a single adenine mutation in 5'UTR of Endothelin-1 gene in paediatric cases with severe pulmonary hypertension: an observational study. BMC Research Notes. 2021;**14**(1):194

[76] Vasku A et al. Interaction of mutations M235T of the gene for angiotensinogen and Taq I 8000 in the gene for endothelin-1 at the onset of essential hypertension. Casopís Lékařů Českých. 2000;**139**(15):464-467

[77] Calabro P, Limongelli G, Maddaloni V, et al. Analysis of endothelin-1 and endothelin-1 receptor A gene polymorphisms in patients with pulmonary arterial hypertension. Internal and Emergency Medicine. 2012;7:425-430

[78] Ferri C, Bellini C, Desideri G, De Mattia G. Endogenous insulin modulates circulating endothelin-1 concentrations in humans. Diabetes Care. 1996;**19**(5): 504-506

[79] Manolio TA et al. Finding the missing heritability of complex diseases. Nature. 2009;**461**(7265):747-753

[80] Eichler EE, Flint J, Gibson G, Kong A, Leal SM, Moore JH, et al. Missing heritability and strategies for finding the underlying causes of complex disease. Nature Reviews. Genetics. 2010;**11**(6):446-450

Chapter 3

Genetic Markers of Endothelial Dysfunction

Iwona Wybranska

Abstract

The rate of endothelial dysfunction is influenced by genetic variation and thus inherited in families. Genetic disorders, such as familial hypercholesterolemia and homocystinuria, are at risk for premature atherosclerosis, and exhibit early endothelial dysfunction. The known spectrum of mutations in LDL receptor, APOB and PCSK9 gene represent the monogenic dominant hypercholesterolemia. An autosomal recessive form of hypercholesterolaemia in the caused by homozygous mutations in the LDL-R adaptor protein. The polygenic hypercholesterolaemia for patients with a clinical diagnosis of FH is based on the cumulative effect of LDL-C-raising alleles with a cumulative effect, in a complex interaction with the environment that leads to an increase in LDL-C, producing an FH-like phenotype and presenting this type of hypercholesterolaemia as a typical complex disease. The various causes of homocysteinaemia like genetic causes include mutations and enzyme deficiencies such as the most frequently mentioned 5, 10-methylenetetrahydrofolate reductase (MTHFR), but also methionine synthase (MS) and cystathionine β-synthase (CβS) but also by deficiencies of folate, vitamin B12 and, to a lesser extent, deficiencies of vitamin B6, which affects methionine metabolism, and leads also to endothelial disfunction in different mechanismms. Mutations in genes coding enzymes in homocysteine metabolism and also in nitric oxide (NO) synthesis, the main vasodilatator is also presented in this chapter. The crucial importance of microRNAs in endothelial physiology following EC-specific inactivation of the enzyme Dicer which is involved in altered expression of key regulators of endothelial function, including endothelial nitric oxide synthase (eNOS), vascular endothelial growth factor receptor 2 (VEGF), interleukin-8, Tie-1 and Tie-2. The new discoveries based on genome-wide screening (GWAS) complement the knowledge of the topic.

Keywords: asymmetric dimethylarginine, endothelial nitric oxide, low density lipoprotein, hypercholesterolaemia, homocysteinaemia, epigenetic regulation, gene polymorphism, association studies

1. Introduction

A healthy vascular endothelium exerts atheroprotective effects through vasoactive mediators such as nitric oxide (NO), prostacyclin and endothelium-derived hyperpolarizing factor (EDHF). The endothelium plays an important role in regulating vasomotor tone and maintaining vascular integrity. Endothelial dysfunction, impaired endothelium-dependent dilation, is a fundamental element in the pathogenesis of cardiovascular disease. There is evidence that as we age, the endothelium is exposed to the deleterious effects of elevated blood pressure and increased levels of cholesterol, glucose, homocysteine, to products of the inflammatory response and to components of cigarette smoke, and these protective properties decrease, leading to a state of endothelial dysfunction [1]. Although endothelial dysfunction is associated with a number of risk factors for atherosclerosis, these risk factors are not the only determinants of endothelial dysfunction. The rate of endothelial dysfunction is influenced by a number of factors that are determined by genetic variation and thus inherited in families. These issues will be addressed in this chapter.

Vascular atherosclerosis, as the most common sign of endothelial dysfunction, usually manifests itself at a later age, although studies of twins and adoptions indicate that this more common form is also partly heritable, although the inheritance is complex, arising from shared environmental exposures (risk factors) and many common gene variants (polymorphisms) with small to moderate effects. Endothelial dysfunction manifested in atherosclerosis also results from single-gene diseases that strongly modify risk factors, such as hypercholesterolemia or hyperhomocysteinuria. Children with certain single-gene disorders, such as homocystinuria and familial hypercholesterolemia, are at risk for premature atherosclerosis, and also exhibit early endothelial dysfunction [2–4].

2. Aging endothelium—mechanisms of endothelial senescence

Endothelial cell senescence is a physiological process of irreversible cell cycle arrest to which various biological stress conditions such as, telomere shortening, DNA damage, reactive oxygen species (ROS) production and mitochondrial dysfunction contribute. Cellular senescence is a process in which vascular cells stop dividing and undergo characteristic phenotypic changes, such as profound changes in chromatin and secretome [5]. Vascular endothelial cell senescence has been found to play a key role in vascular aging, leading to the initiation, progression and development of vascular atherosclerosis [6]. Aging vascular endothelial cells typically become flatter and enlarged with increasingly polypoid nuclei. These changes are accompanied by modulation of cytoskeletal integrity, angiogenesis, cell proliferation and migration [7]. Aging endothelial cells exhibit decreased production of endothelial nitric oxide (NO), increased release of endothelin-1 (ET-1), increased inflammation and cell apoptosis [7]. Senescence of endothelial cells thus induces structural and functional changes in blood vessels, exacerbating thrombosis, inflammation and atherosclerosis with impaired vascular tone, angiogenesis and vascular integrity, which contributes to the development and progression of atherosclerosis [8]. However, the molecular mechanisms of vascular endothelial cell aging and their relationship to underlying pathophysiological changes are not yet fully understood. In this chapter, the role of genetic factors affecting the mechanisms of endothelial cell senescence in the process of vascular aging and the development of atherosclerosis will be discussed.

Cellular senescence is a physiological or pathological process that occurs throughout life [9]. Under physiological conditions, cellular senescence is involved in embryonic tissue development, tissue repair, and tumor suppression responses [9]. However, the accumulation of senescent cells can lead to loss of replicative capacity, cell apoptosis, unfavorable structural changes and the associated development of atherosclerosis [9]. Cellular senescence is usually associated with aging and age-related disorders. In human coronary arteries, endothelial cells with increased β-galactosidase activity associated with enhanced senescence are observed during aging, suggesting that aging is also associated with decreased endothelial cell regeneration and endothelial cell senescence, which is associated with decreased endothelium-dependent arterial relaxation [10] and the development of arterial stiffness [9]. Several studies have found that NO donors reduce arterial stiffness in healthy subjects and in patients with hypertension and hypercholesterolemia [10]. These data support a role for aging vascular endothelial cells in the pathogenesis of arteriosclerosis. However, while few clinical studies have examined the relationship between endothelial aging, arterial stiffness and hypertension, those that have been conducted have shown that aging is closely associated with arterial stiffness and atherosclerosis. For example, data from the Framingham Heart Study showed that older age was significantly associated with higher carotid-femoral pulse wave velocity and mean arterial pressure [11]. Arterial stiffness has been shown to be an independent biomarker of atherosclerotic morbidity and mortality in the general population, in aging individuals, in patients with hypertension and in patients with end-stage renal disease [12]. With aging and the associated arterial stiffness, systolic blood pressure tends to increase while diastolic blood pressure tends to decrease, and this pathophysiological change results in an increase in pulse pressure and pulse wave velocity in the aorta. Indeed, it has also been observed that the prevalence of hypertension, especially isolated systolic hypertension, is increased in the aging population [13]. Increased systolic pressure increases left ventricular afterload with an associated increase in myocardial oxygen demand. Declining diastolic pressure reduces perfusion of the coronary circulation during diastole. These consequences of arterial stiffness, increased systolic pressure and decreased diastolic pressure further induce left ventricular hypertrophy and subsequent myocardial ischaemia, remodeling and other cardiovascular complications in aging individuals [8].

3. Cholesterol—factor of endothelial senescence and endothelial dysfunction

Senescence of endothelial cells is known to mediate the endothelial damage that occurs during the initial phase of atherosclerosis. Aging cells of the vascular wall lead to endothelial dysfunction, resulting in the synthesis of inflammatory cytokines and promoting the progression of atherosclerosis. The second stage of developing atherosclerosis, fibrous plaque formation, is characterized by increased lipid accumulation in the intima, resulting in fibrous tissue proliferation and vitreous degeneration, forming characteristic plaques in the intima. Also, macrophages accumulate in the subendothelial space, where they induce pathology by increasing the expression of key atherogenic and inflammatory cytokines and chemokines [14]. In the third stage, atherosclerotic plaque formation, the fibrous tissue is large and necrotic, enriched in lipids, while the lesion surface is thinner and few foam cells are present at the base and margin. In atherosclerotic lesions, smooth muscle cells of the vascular wall migrate from the media to the intima, accumulate around the lipid core formed by dead foam cells and switch from a contractile to a synthetic phenotype. Macrophages, on the other hand, which phagocytized lipids, display an abnormal or activated phenotype, which promotes pathological vascular proliferation [15]. At this stage, proliferation dominates the smooth muscle cells of the vascular wall, but aging does not occur and a typical atherosclerotic plaque is formed. The fourth stage involves changes secondary to atherosclerotic plaques, in which aging macrophages promote plaque instability, degradation of elastic fibers and thinning of the fibrous cap, as well as increased expression of metalloproteases and formation of ulcers and thrombi [14]. At this stage, foam cells induce senescence of human vascular endothelial cells by releasing 4-hydroxynonenal (4-HNE) [16], which exacerbates senescence and induces atherosclerosis. Senescent human vascular wall smooth muscle cells differentiate into an osteogenic phenotype and undergo expression of calcifying factors, which eventually leads to calcification of the atherosclerotic plaque. It is noteworthy that human vascular smooth muscle cells proliferate in the early phase of atherosclerotic plaque formation. However, the proliferation rate of these cells is lower in advanced plaques than in early lesions, indicating that cell senescence may occur [17]. In addition, vascular injury and phenotypic transformation of senescent human vascular wall smooth muscle cells also play a role in mediating vascular calcification [18]. Cellular aging is not a consequence of a single cause, but there are many factors that can induce cellular aging. Premature cellular aging, can be caused by factors such as miRNAs, homocysteine, hyperglycaemia, hypertension, hyperlipidaemia, hyperphosphataemia and oxidative stress, by reducing telomerase activity, increasing ROS production and promoting vascular calcification, mitochondrial dysfunction and DNA damage.

High cholesterol and triglyceride levels have also been found to be associated with an increased risk of atherosclerosis and shorter life expectancy. In fact, the vascular endothelial dysfunction that occurs during human aging is the factor, and the accumulation of lipids in the vascular endothelium activates leukocytes to produce cytokines and chemokines that recruit macrophages. On the other hand, macrophages enhance the inflammatory response and secrete vascular endothelial growth factor, a key cytokine that mediates angiogenesis and the inflammatory response. And hyperlipidaemia itself is a major risk factor for aging, hypertension and diabetes.

The relationship between hypercholesterolemia, atherosclerosis and aging is still poorly understood. Low-density lipoprotein (LDL) (cholesterol) in general is an important physiological compound for cellular function, but in high concentrations can lead to atherosclerosis. It is generally accepted that the oxidized form of cholesterol leads to endothelial dysfunction, which is the initial step in the formation of atherosclerotic plaques. Oxidized low-density lipoprotein acts by binding to multiple scavenger receptors (SRs), such as SR-AI, SR-A2, and can also increase the expression of endothelial cells' own LOX-Ion receptor and activate these cells [19–21]. Under physiological conditions, endothelial cells secrete many factors, monitor the transport of plasma molecules and regulate vascular tone. In addition, endothelial cells are involved in the regulation of cholesterol and lipid homeostasis, signal transduction, immunity and inflammation [22]. And, in addition, oxidized low-density lipoprotein promotes the growth and migration of smooth muscle cells, fibroblasts and macrophages. Vascular lesions are most often caused by hypercholesterolaemia, which can be induced by dietary supplementation, overproduction of lipoproteins by the liver or genetic mutations of lipid receptors and other proteins that regulate lipid homeostatic pathways.

3.1 Mutations of genes regulating the cholesterol level

Hypercholesterolaemia is a common, and still underdiagnosed, autosomal dominantly inherited disorder that is estimated to occur at a prevalence of ≈1 in 220 people worldwide. Familial hypercholesterolaemia (FH) is characterized by a persistent lifelong elevation of low-density lipoprotein cholesterol (LDL-C) and, if untreated, leads to early onset atherosclerosis and an increased risk of cardiovascular events. Untreated hypercholesterolaemia in men and women is associated with a very high risk ranging from 30–50% of having a fatal or non-fatal cardiac event at 50 and 60 years of age, respectively [23]. The most common cause of single-gene familial hypercholesterolaemia is pathogenic variants in the LDL receptor gene (LDL-R), which account for 85–90% of genetically confirmed cases of familial FH. Pathogenic variants in the gene for apolipoprotein (ApoB), a ligand for the LDL receptor, a component of LDL resulting in reduced binding of LDL to LDL-R, or gain-of-function mutations in the gene for proprotein convertase subtilisin/kexin 9 (PCSK9), resulting in increased destruction of LDL-R, account for 5–15% and 1% of cases of monogenic hypercholesterolaemia, respectively [24]. There is also an autosomal recessive form of hypercholesterolaemia in the human population, caused by homozygous mutations in the LDL-R adaptor protein which, is associated with the mild phenotype of homozygous hypercholesterolaemia found in Sardinian residents [25].

With the exception of the homozygous form of familial hypercholesterolemia (HoFH), FH is generally a silent disease. HoFH usually manifests with pathognomonic physical symptoms in childhood, such as cantelosis, tendon xanthoma and corneal arching. FH is diagnosed clinically based on a weighted combination of physical findings, personal or family history of hypercholesterolemia, early ischemic disease in the family and circulating LDL-C levels. The genetic cause is highly heterogeneous. Mutations in the LDL receptor genome are very common and occur at different sites disrupting receptor function in different ways. They therefore have different pathological significance. The spectrum of functional alterations in APOB outside the fragments routinely screened is growing. The ClinVar database at NCBI shows all the mutations in this gene described to date. There are about 3000 of them, and of these mutations that are labeled as pathological there are about 1000. They are mainly missense, nonsense frameshift mutations including about 500 deletions and 170 duplications. The largest number of known mutations are single nucleotide mutations mainly in coding regions of the gene, about 2000.

The known spectrum of mutations in APOB has been increasing in recent years thanks to next-generation sequencing (NGS) techniques, which allow all 29 exons of APOB to be studied without increasing laboratory workload [26–29]. However, as APOB is a highly polymorphic gene, these variants require functional assessment before a clear diagnosis can be made [27]. It is also known that mutations in the APOB gene do not have 100 per cent penetrance, and the phenotype of patients is usually milder than in patients with FH caused by LDLR mutations [30].

The ClinVar database from NCBI is being updated with known pathological mutations in the APOB gene. There are currently 84 of them, most of which are located in the hydrophilic part of the apoB protein, the part that can bind to the LDL receptor. Mutations of the nonsense, missense and reading frame shift types dominate among the pathologies leading to familial hypercholesterolemia.

Familial hypercholesterolemia (FH), a major risk factor for coronary artery disease (CAD), is typically caused by mutations in genes that code for proteins responsible for removing low density lipoprotein (LDL) from the circulation. Only 17 pathogenic mutations in the PCSK9 gene are currently known and presented in the ClinVar database from NCBI. PCSK9 was discovered in 2003 when gain-of-function (GOF) mutations in this gene were identified as causative of FH in an autosomal dominant manner [31]. These GOF mutations are associated with hypercholesterolemia and a higher risk of CAD [32–36]. For example, a mutation in the apoB gene p.S127R is specifically associated with overproduction of this protein, resulting in greater synthesis of very low-density lipoprotein (VLDL), intermediate-density lipoprotein

(IDL) and, consequently, LDL [32]. Another mutation of this gene p.E670G is associated more with serum lipid parameters, including total cholesterol (TC), high-density lipoprotein (HDL) and Apo B [33], as well as with an increased risk of stroke due to large vessel atherosclerosis and ischaemic stroke [36]. Serum PCSK9 levels, has been identified as a major predictor of carotid atherosclerosis independent of other risk factors in asymptomatic patients [37]. Furthermore, the contribution of PCSK9 concentrations to FH severity appears to be independent of LDL receptor genotype [38]. Recently, a homozygous gain-of-function mutation of the PCSK9 gene was characterized that is associated with the phenotype of a patient whose cholesterol is 316 mg/dl and LDL was 234 mg/dl at the age of 11 years [39]. This patient has no mutations in the LDL receptor or Apo B genes [39].

Loss-of-function mutations of the PCSK9 gene are associated with hypocholesterolaemia and significant protection against CAD [40–43]. Notably, the p.Y142X mutation is found only in 0.4 per cent of African Americans, but not in other ethnic groups [40]. The p.C679X mutation is more common in African Americans and Zimbabwean Africans, but very rare in European Americans [41]. One individual has been described who is homozygous for the p.R46L mutation and has a total cholesterol level of 11 mg/dl [42]. In one family, six of the eight members who carry the p.R46L mutation have LDL levels below the bottom 10% percentile of LDL [42]. Another study reported that two healthy women with 'loss of function' mutations affecting both alleles of the PCSK9 gene have extremely low LDL cholesterol levels (14 mg/dL) [41–43].

The concept of polygenic hypercholesterolaemia for patients with a clinical diagnosis of FH but no monogenic cause was presented in 2013 by Talmud et al. [44]. This concept is based on the cumulative effect of LDL-C-raising alleles with a cumulative effect, perhaps in a complex interaction with the environment that leads to an increase in LDL-C, producing an FH-like phenotype and presenting this type of hypercholesterolaemia as a typical complex disease.

The more often publishing genes with polymorphisms contributing to the high cholesterol phenotype include cadherin EGF LAG 7-pass G-type receptor 2, ATP-binding cassette subfamily G members 5 & 8 (ABCG5/8), sterol regulatory element binding protein-2 (SREBP-2), signal transducing adaptor family member 1 (STAP1), and Apo E. Talmud's group developed a genetic risk score (GRS) based on scoring 12 SNPs where individuals above the top decile of the distribution of LDL-C scores were described as having a higher probability of polygenic hypercholesterolaemia [44]. Then, by removing SNPs with smaller effects/lower frequencies, they showed that a weighted score of six SNPs performed as well as a score of 12-SNPs. The top three quartiles of the distribution also indicated a greater likelihood of a polygenic explanation for their elevated LDL-C [45]. Another study established the 10-SNP GRS, which showed a strong association with high LDL cholesterol, confirming the validity of this score as a genetic risk marker for elevated LDL cholesterol [46]. In this cohort, individuals with an extreme weighted GRS $\geq$1.96 ($\geq$90th percentile) were defined as having polygenic severe hypercholesterolaemia. Research has gone further and a study of patients with severe hypercholesterolaemia found that a high polygenic score for 2 million-SNP LDL-C (upper 5th percentile) could explain hypercholesterolaemia in up to 23% of patients, while only 2% carried a monogenic mutation [47].

With the development of genetic testing in recent years, a mutation in any of the three known autosomal dominant genes causing familial hypercholesterolaemia is found in the majority of cases with a clinical diagnosis of familial hypercholesterolaemia. SituationBecause individuals with polygenic background hypercholesterolaemia do not have the same inheritance pattern observed in monogenic familial hypercholesterolaemia, familial cascade screening is not recommended for individuals with polygenic background, as only 30% of relatives have elevated LDL-C levels compared to 50% in monogenic families. The presence of a causative monogenic mutation is associated with the highest cardiovascular risk vs. no mutation or polygenic ancestry, providing prognostic information independent of LDL-C. This may also help to assess the intensity of intervention. Treatment adherence also appears to be higher after monogenic confirmation of hypercholesterolaemia.

4. Homocystein—factor of endothelial senescence and endothelial dysfunction

In addition to cholesterol, the second important factor whose high blood concentration causes vascular endothelial damage is homocysteine. Homocysteine (Hcy) is a sulfur-containing non-proteinogenic amino acid formed during the metabolism of the essential amino acid methionine. Hcy is considered an independent risk factor for atherosclerosis and cardiovascular disease, but the molecular basis of these compounds remains incompletely elucidated to date. There is a causal link, as studies have observed that impaired endothelial function, a key initial event in the development of atherosclerosis and CVD, is observed in hyperhomocysteinemia (HHcy). Various phenomena may explain the vascular toxicity associated with high homocysteine concentrations. For example, Hcy is an inhibitor of nitric oxide (NO) synthesis, a gaseous master regulator of endothelial homeostasis. In addition, Hcy is responsible for deregulating the signaling pathways associated with hydrogen sulphide another important endothelial gasotransmitter. Hcy is also involved in the loss of critical endothelial antioxidant systems and thus increases the intracellular concentration of reactive oxygen species (ROS) causing oxidative stress. ROS interfere with lipoprotein metabolism, forming oxidized forms of lipids that are removed by vascular wall macrophages contributing to the development of atherosclerotic vascular lesions. In addition, excess Hcy can be indirectly incorporated into proteins, a process referred to as N-homocysteinylation of proteins, inducing vascular damage. The inability to metabolize homocysteine and excess homocysteine decreases the synthesis of the universal methyl group donor, so necessary for epigenetic processes occurring in cells, and the hypomethylation of cellular DNA caused by the accumulation of S-adenosylhomocysteine (AdoHcy) also contributes to the molecular basis of Hcy-induced vascular toxicity and endothelial cell aging. A negative regulator of cellular methyltransferases, AdoHcy is a metabolic precursor of Hcy that accumulates under HHcy conditions [48].

4.1 Genetics of homocysteinaemia

There are various causes of homocysteinaemia. Genetic causes include mutations and enzyme deficiencies such as the most frequently mentioned 5, 10-methylene-tetrahydrofolate reductase (MTHFR), but also methionine synthase (MS) and cystathionine β-synthase (CβS). In addition, HHcy can be caused by a diet rich in folate, but also by deficiencies of folate, vitamin B12 and, to a lesser extent, deficiencies of vitamin B6, which affects methionine metabolism, and also by impaired renal function.

MTHFR catalyzes the conversion reaction of 5,10-methylenetetrahydrofolate to 5-methyltetrahydrofolate, which is an intermediate in the conversion of Hcy to methionine. Mutations in MTHFR occur frequently in the population and are common inborn errors of folate metabolism that result in phenotypes ranging from asymptomatic to severe neurological deterioration and even early death in the classic form of MTHFR deficiency [49].

Homocystinuria is also an autosomal recessive error of metabolism resulting from defects in the cobalamin (vitamin B12)-dependent pathway that converts Hcy to methionine and is catalyzed by the enzyme methionine synthase.

Hcy in the blood is generally found 70–80% as a disulfide bound to plasma proteins, 20–30% as a homodimer with itself and about 1% as a free thiol, or a heterodimer with other thiols [50]. Levels of the Hcy are usually controlled by 2 biochemical processes: (1) roughly ~50% of the Hcy goes to transsulfuration pathway for producing the glutathione and the remaining and (2) ~50% can be remethylated back to methionine [51, 52]. Normally, the synthesis and elimination of Hcy stay pretty much in balance, but in diseased conditions, i.e., in HHcy, the overall plasma Hcy levels tend to increase due to the errors in the Hcy metabolism [53].

Causes of homocystinaemia include regular consumption of an excessively methionine-rich protein diet, or B12/folate deficiency, or 'loss-of-function type' mutations of the CBS gene as heterozygous or homozygous, and finally insufficient Hcy clearance from the kidney. Several other factors are influential among which are gender, age, smoking, alcohol consumption, certain medications, and medical conditions that can potentially modulate the methionine cycle can increase Hcy levels. Furthermore, there are additional genetic factors that are key in promoting HHcy status, such as genetic defects in enzyme proteins involved in '1-carbon metabolism' [54–56]. As this cycle is the only pathway that gives methyl group in both biosynthesis of cellular compounds such as creatine, epinephrine, carnitine, phospholipids, proteins, and polyamines and in epigenetic changes (like methylation of DNA, RNA, and histones) [57]. Nevertheless, HHcy mediated metabolic malfunctioning because of the higher circulating Hcy levels promote oxidant stress-induced vascular inflammation and vessel dysfunction leading to atherosclerosis, myocardial infarction, stroke, multiple sclerosis, cognitive impairment, epilepsy, dementia, Parkinson's disease, and ocular disorders [58, 59].

An interesting scientific discussion is being conducted in the context of the importance of the common MTHFR gene polymorphism and its significance in endothelial diseases. Heterozygous polymorphisms of the MTHFR gene reduce enzyme activity by 40% (CT variant, MTHFR c. [665C > T];[665C =]) and up to 70% in the homozygous form (TT variant, MTHFR c. [665C > T], [665C > T]). The CT variant is very common as it occurs in up to 20–40% of the Caucasian population and 1–4% of most other ethnic groups. The homozygous TT variant occurs in about 10% of the general population in Europe.

Retrospective studies conducted in the 1980s showed an increased prevalence of homocysteine concentrations in the 15–30 μmol/l range dependent on the MTHFR 677C > T polymorphism (new nomenclature, c.665 C > T) in the presence of concomitant folate deficiency in patients with atherosclerosis after myocardial infarction, stroke and coronary artery disease, and with a history of venous thromboembolism (VTE), i.e. deep vein thrombosis and/or pulmonary embolism. Quite different results were published from a prospective study published in 2002 in which these correlations were shown to be weak or even non-existent. In 2010, the American College of Cardiology and the American Heart Association unequivocally spoke out against homocysteine determination in cardiovascular risk assessment, considering hyperhomocysteinaemia to be a non-significant risk factor at the public health level [60].

In contrast, during protein biosynthesis, Hcy can be misused by methionyl-tRNA synthase to produce homocysteine thiolactone (HTL), a cyclic thioester that reacts rapidly with proteins to form amide bonds with the amino groups of lysine residues [61]. The resulting N-homocysteinylated proteins with altered structure and biochemical properties contribute to the vascular pathology associated with HHcy [62]. In fact, studies on cell cultures confirmed that Hcy supplemented in the medium was converted to HTL, and the extent of this conversion was proportional to Hcy concentration.

5. Gene polymorphisms influencing vasomotor endothelial function

Nitric oxide (NO), is a key vasodilator. It is formed in the vascular endothelium by the oxidation of arginine through the catalytic activity of nitric oxide synthase (NOS). This reaction requires NADPH and O2 as co-substrate and yields NO and citrulline as end products. Importantly, the enzymatic activity of NOS is inhibited by methylated analogues of arginine, namely N-monomethylarginine (L-NMMA) and asymmetric dimethylarginine (ADMA) [63], which are synthesized in vivo by a family of enzymes known as protein arginine methyltransferases. Proteolysis of proteins containing L-NMMA and ADMA releases them into the endothelial cell cytosol, from where they are removed into the blood. Elevated serum ADMA levels are associated with atherosclerotic vascular disease [64].

More than 15 polymorphisms exist in the NOS3 promoter that might influence mRNA transcription and reduce gene expression. Two polymorphisms in NOS3, 786 T > C and 894G > T, are the most studied. 786 T > C resides in the promoter region of NOS3 and regulates transcriptional initiation [65]. However, the –786 T > C polymorphism has shown inconsistent associations with functional measures, and with clinical disease end points. The CC genotype at 786 T > C is associated with blunted forearm blood flow responses to Ach in hypertensive subjects [66] and no increases in NOS3 mRNA and endothelial nitric oxide synthase (eNOS) protein expression in response to laminar shear stress in endothelial cells from coronary heart patients [67]. Polymorphisms within the coding region of the NOS 3 gene could alter NOS enzymatic activity. The 894G > T polymorphism in exon 7 of NOS3 results in substitution of glutamate with aspartate at codon 298 (also denoted as Glu298Asp) [68]. There is currently a debate, with controversial studies on whether this polymorphism is indeed functional. Two studies have shown that eNOS Asp298 undergoes selective proteolytic cleavage in endothelial cells and vascular tissues, which may account for reduced vascular NO production [69]. However, other studies have suggested that this finding may be the result of an artifact [70].

ADMA is removed from the circulation by metabolism primarily by isoform two of the DDAH2 dimethylarginine dimethylaminohydrolase, which predominates in tissues that express eNOS, such as the endothelium. The main cause of elevated ADMA levels in patients at risk for vascular disease is not fully understood, but one potential explanation could be loss-of-function mutations in the DDAH enzyme gene that alter gene expression or enzyme activity. Six potentially pathological polymorphisms have been identified in the DDAH2 gene. Five of them are upstream of the translation start site and may affect gene transcription. An insertion-deletion polymorphism (6G/7G) at position 2871, which lies in the core promoter region, affected DDAH2 promoter activity in the promoter/reporter assay [71].

The realization that common gene variants can, at best, have little to moderate impact on physiology and disease susceptibility has led to the understanding that future studies of susceptibility to complex diseases, whether they address clinical endpoints or intermediate phenotypes such as endothelial function, will need to be much larger and include more variables simultaneously. Because many GWAS identify SNPs outside protein coding regions or in non-coding intervals, the contribution of small non-coding RNA (e.g., lncRNA, microRNA) in modulating endothelial function should be addressed.

6. Micro-RNA and its epigenetic role in endothelial pathophysiology

Indisputably, microRNAs are fundamental regulators of many biological processes. Regulation of basic vascular endothelial functions by microRNAs and its disruption can lead to endothelial dysfunction. MicroRNAs are small, generally non-coding RNAs that regulate the expression of many genes through post-transcriptional degradation or translational repression. The crucial importance of microRNAs in endothelial physiology has been demonstrated following EC-specific inactivation of the enzyme Dicer which is involved in the biogenesis and processing of microRNAs, which cleaves microRNA precursors into mature forms [72, 73]. The absence of Dicer in the endothelium leads to altered expression of key regulators of endothelial function, including endothelial nitric oxide synthase (eNOS), vascular endothelial growth factor receptor 2 (VEGF), interleukin-8, Tie-1 and Tie-2.

Recent studies have identified miR-19a as an important driver of upregulation of important factors implicated in endothelial dysfunction, hyperlipidemia, inflammation and atherosclerosis, revealing a vicious cycle involving endothelial Hif-1a activation, hyperlipidemia and upregulation of miR-19a, promoting CXCR2 (C-X-C Motif Chemokine Receptor 2 which mediates neutrophil migration to sites of inflammation) dependent monocyte adhesion by increasing endothelial expression of its ligand CXCL1 [74]. It is also worth noting that microRNAs are also involved in switching the phenotype of VSMCs between a quiescent (pro-contractile, differentiated) and proliferative (pro-synthetic, differentiated) state [75], a critical step in the pathophysiology of atherosclerosis.

The endothelium has a critical role in maintaining vascular integrity and protecting against cardiovascular disease. Accumulated data indicate endothelial function is a heritable trait regulated by polygenic factors; however, these genetic factors have not been fully elucidated until now.

7. New discoveries based on genome-wide screening (GWAS)

Genome-wide association studies (GWAS) have been widely used in recent years to identify new genetic loci underlying chronic diseases. GWAS for endothelial function have been relatively limited due to the different phenotypes associated with it. The first such study was conducted by Vasan and colleagues for several cardiovascular traits, including FMD (%) and hyperemic flow velocity in 1345 individuals from the Framingham Heart Study, using a set of 100kSNPs [76]. They identified several SNPs associated with each trait in this study, including chloride channel (CFTR) and phosphodiesterase 5A (PDE5A) SNPs. Although these results have not been replicated, this was the first GWAS to directly examine endothelial function on a large population.

Yoshino and colleagues conducted an association study on the coronary vascular response to acetylcholine (ACh), a common index of coronary endothelial function, in 643 female and male subjects [77]. They used a set of 1536 SNPs located in genes related to cardiovascular physiology and pathology. The results showed that variants in adenosine A1 receptor (ADORA1) were associated with endothelial dysfunction in the entire cohort, while variants in adenosine A3 receptor (ADORA3) and lipoprotein(a) (LPA) had the strongest associations with increased risk of endothelial dysfunction in women only.

In recent genome-wide association study (GWAS) studies in European population, three novel sites related to endothelial dysfunction were found [78, 79]: Vascular endothelial growth factor A (VEGFA) rs9472135, Faciogenital dysplasia 5 (FGD5) rs11128722, Zinc Finger C3HC-type Containing 1 (ZC3HC1) rs11556924.

Because many GWAS identify SNPs outside protein coding regions or in non-coding intervals, the contribution of small non-coding RNA (e.g., lncRNA, microRNA) in modulating endothelial function should be addressed. In 2011, genome-wide association studies (GWAS) identified ANRIL as a biomarker closely associated with coronary heart disease (CHD) [80]. These studies identified, locus 9p21 which contains many single nucleotide polymorphisms (SNPs) that are located in a "gene desert" without any protein-coding genes. A key portion of the SNPs at the 9p21 locus overlap with six exons in the ANRIL gene also known as CDKN2B-AS or CDKN2B-AS1, which is transcribed in the antisense direction in the INK4b-ARF-INK4a gene cluster. ANRIL is expressed in vascular endothelial cells, vascular smooth muscle cells, mononuclear phagocytes and atherosclerotic plaques and its variation is associated with vascular endothelial malfunction, vascular smooth muscle cell (VSMC) including proliferation, migration, senescence, apoptosis, mononuclear cell adhesion and proliferation, glycolipid metabolism disorders and DNA damage [81].

Heritable changes in gene activity and expression also can be the result of epigenetic changes. Recent evidence suggests epigenetic changes such as those induced by histonemethyltransferase Set7 are associated with endothelial dysfunction, including impaired FMD in diabetics [82].

The problem with the paucity of GWAS studies is that most disease-relevant single nucleotide polymorphisms (SNPs) cannot be assigned to a specific gene, and even demonstrating that a single SNP affects gene expression is not possible for most SNPs. This is a consequence of the complex architecture of the genome, in which enhancers are often located far from their target gene in a two-dimensional sequence-based projection. The second aspect is a consequence of the heterocellularity of the atherosclerotic lesion, such that a specific SNP is relevant in only one of the many different cell types expressed in the lesion.

In the future, thanks to the already initiated GWAS studies in single cells of the atherosclerotic lesion, this second problem may be solved.

Author details

Iwona Wybranska
Department of Clinical Biochemistry, Genetics and Nutrigenomics, Chair of Clinical Biochemistry, The Jagiellonian University Medical Collage, Krakow, Poland

*Address all correspondence to: iwona.wybranska@uj.edu.pl

IntechOpen

© 2023 The Author(s). Licensee IntechOpen. This chapter is distributed under the terms of the Creative Commons Attribution License (http://creativecommons.org/licenses/by/3.0), which permits unrestricted use, distribution, and reproduction in any medium, provided the original work is properly cited.

References

[1] Vallance P, Chan N. Endothelial function and nitric oxide: Clinical relevance. Heart. 2001;**85**:342-350

[2] Celermajer DS, Sorensen K, Ryalls M, et al. Impaired endothelial function occurs in the systemic arteries of children with homozygous homocystinuria but not in their heterozygous parents. Journal of the American College of Cardiology. 1993;**22**:854-858

[3] Celermajer DS, Sorensen KE, Gooch VM, et al. Non-invasive detection of endothelial dysfunction in children and adults at risk of atherosclerosis. Lancet. 1992;**340**:1111-1115

[4] Marenberg ME, Risch N, Berkman LF, et al. Genetic susceptibility to death from coronary heart disease in a study of twins. The New England Journal of Medicine. 1994;**330**:1041-1046

[5] Rossman MJ, Kaplon RE, Hill SD, McNamara MN, Santos-Parker JR, Pierce GL, et al. Endothelial cell senescence with aging in healthy humans: Prevention by habitual exercise and relation to vascular endothelial. American Journal of Physiology. Heart and Circulatory Physiology. 2017;**313**:H890-H895. DOI: 10.1152/ajpheart.00416.2017

[6] Hohensinner PJ, Kaun C, Buchberger E, Ebenbauer B, Demyanets S, Huk I, et al. Age intrinsic loss of telomere protection via TRF1 reduction in endothelial cells Biochim. Biochimica et Biophysica Acta. 1863;**2016**:360-367

[7] Uryga AK, Bennett MR. Ageing induced vascular smooth muscle cell senescence in atherosclerosis. The Journal of Physiology. 2016;**594**:2115-2124

[8] Jia G, Aroor AR, DeMarco VG, Martinez-Lemus LA, Meininger GA, Sowers JR. Vascular stiffness in insulin resistance and obesity. Frontiers in Physiology. 2015;**6**:231

[9] He S, Sharpless NE. Senescence in health and disease. Cell. 2017;**169**:1000-1011

[10] Liu JH, Chen Y, Zhen Z, Yeung CK, Chan J, Chan HH, et al. Relation between endothelial progenitor cells and arterial stiffness in patients with psoriasis. The Journal of Dermatology. 2016;**43**:888-893

[11] Mitchell GF, Parise H, Benjamin EJ, Larson MG, Keyes MJ, Vita JA, et al. Changes in arterial stiffness and wave reflection with advancing age in healthy men and women: The Framingham heart study. Hypertension. 2004;**43**:1239-1245

[12] Mitchell GF, Hwang SJ, Vasan RS, Larson MG, Pencina MJ, Hamburg NM, et al. Arterial stiffness and cardiovascular events: The Framingham heart study. Circulation. 2010;**121**:505-511

[13] Vasan RS, Beiser A, Seshadri S, Larson MG, Kannel WB, D'Agostino RB, et al. Residual lifetime risk for developing hypertension in middle-aged women and men: The Framingham heart study. The Journal of the American Medical Association. 2002;**287**:1003-1010

[14] Childs BG, Baker DJ, Wijshake T, Conover CA, Campisi J, Deursen MV. Senescent intimal foam cells are deleterious at all stages of atherosclerosis. Scientometrics. 2016;**354**:472-477. DOI: 10.1126/science.aaf6659

[15] Sene A, Khan AA, Cox D, Nakamura REI, Santeford A, Kim BM, et al. Impaired cholesterol efflux in

senescent macrophages promotes age-related macular degeneration. Cell Metabolism. 2013;**17**:549-561. DOI: 10.1016/j.cmet.2013.03.009

[16] Riahi Y, Kaiser N, Cohen G, Abd-Elrahman I, Blum G, Shapira OM, et al. Foam cell-derived 4-hydroxynonenal induces endothelial cell senescence in a TXNIP-dependent manner. Journal of Cellular and Molecular Medicine. 2015;**19**:1887-1899. DOI: 10.1111/jcmm.12561

[17] Bennett MR, Macdonald K, Chan SW, Boyle JJ, Weissberg PL. Cooperative interactions between RB and p53 regulate cell proliferation, cell senescence, and apoptosis in human vascular smooth muscle cells from atherosclerotic plaques. Circulation Research. 1998;**82**:704-712. DOI: 10.1161/01.res.82.6.704

[18] Bonomini F, Taurone S, Parnigotto P, Zamai L, Rodella LF, Artico M, et al. Role of parnaparin in atherosclerosis. International Journal of Experimental Pathology. 2016;**97**:457-464. DOI: 10.1111/iep.12217

[19] Draude G, Hrboticky N, Lorenz RL. The expression of the lectin-like oxidized low-density lipoprotein receptor (LOX-I) on human vascular smooth muscle cells and monocytes and its down-regulation by lovastatin. Biochemical Pharmacology. 1999;**57**:383-386

[20] Tripodi D, D'Ercole S, Pasini M, Nastasio S, Bonini S, Giuca MR. Inflammatory and immunitary modifications in saliva of subjects with labial and tongue piercing. European Journal of Inflammation. 2011;**9**:185-191

[21] Mirzaei K, Hossein-Nezhad A, Mokhtari F, Najmafshar A, Khoshniat NM. VISFATINI NAMPTIPBCEF and cytokine concentration in multiple sclerosis patients compared to healthy subjects. European Journal of Inflammation. 2011;**9**:31-37

[22] Mehta D, Malik AB. Signaling mechanisms regulating endothelial permeability. Physiological Reviews. 2006;**86**:279-367

[23] Sturm AC, Knowles JW, Gidding SS, Ahmad ZS, Ahmed CD, Ballantyne CM, et al. Convened by the familial hypercholesterolemia foundation. Clinical genetic testing for familial hypercholesterolemia: JACC scientific expert panel. Journal of the American College of Cardiology. 2018;**72**:662-680

[24] Soutar AK, Naoumova RP. Mechanisms of disease: Genetic causes of familial hypercholesterolemia. Nature Clinical Practice. Cardiovascular Medicine. 2007;**4**:214-225

[25] Cuchel M, Bruckert E, Ginsberg HN, Raal FJ, Santos RD, Hegele RA, et al. European Atherosclerosis Society Consensus Panel on Familial Hypercholesterolaemia. Homozygous familial hypercholesterolaemia: New insights and guidance for clinicians to improve detection and clinical management. A position paper from the Consensus Panel on Familial Hypercholesterolaemia of the European Atherosclerosis Society. European Heart Journal. 2014;**35**:2146-2157

[26] Motazacker MM, Pirruccello J, Huijgen R, Do R, Gabriel S, Peter J, et al. Advances in genetics show the need for extending screening strategies for autosomal dominant hypercholesterolaemia. European Heart Journal. 2012;**33**:1360-1366. DOI: 10.1093/eurheartj/ehs010

[27] Alves AC, Etxebarria A, Soutar AK, Martin C, Bourbon M. Novel

functional APOB mutations outside LDL-binding region causing familial hypercholesterolaemia. Human Molecular Genetics and Genomics. 2014;**23**:1817-1828. DOI: 10.1093/hmg/ddt573

[28] Thomas ERA, Atanur SS, Norsworthy PJ, Encheva V, Snijders AP, Game L, et al. Identification and biochemical analysis of a novel APOB mutation that causes autosomal dominant hypercholesterolemia Mol. Molecular Genetics & Genomic Medicine. 2013;**1**:155-161. DOI: 10.1002/mgg3.17

[29] Myant NB. Familial defective apolipoprotein B-100: A review, including some comparisons with familial hypercholesterolaemia. Atherosclerosis. 1993;**104**:1-18

[30] Vrablík M, Ceska R, Horínek A. Major apolipoprotein B-100 mutations in lipoprotein metabolism and atherosclerosis. Physiological Research. 2001;**50**:337-343

[31] Abifadel M, Varret M, Rabes JP, Allard D, Ouguerram K, Devillers M, et al. Mutations in PCSK9 cause autosomal dominant hypercholesterolemia. Nature Genetics. 2003;**34**:154-156

[32] Abifadel M, Guerin M, Benjannet S, Rabes JP, Le Goff W, Julia Z, et al. Identification and characterization of new gain-of-function mutations in the PCSK9 gene responsible for autosomal dominant hypercholesterolemia. Atherosclerosis. 2012;**223**:394-400

[33] Ouguerram K, Chetiveaux M, Zair Y, Costet P, Abifadel M, Varret M, et al. Apolipoprotein B100 metabolism in autosomal-dominanthypercholesterolemia related to mutations in PCSK9. Arteriosclerosis, Thrombosis, and Vascular Biology. 2004;**24**:1448-1453

[34] Abboud S, Karhunen PJ, Lutjohann D, Goebeler S, Luoto T, Friedrichs S, et al. Proprotein convertase subtilisin/Kexin type 9 (PCSK9) gene is a risk factor of large-vessel atherosclerosis stroke. PLoS One. 2007;**2**:e1043

[35] Norata GD, Garlaschelli K, Grigore L, Raselli S, Tramontana S, Meneghetti F, et al. Effects of PCSK9 variants on common carotid artery intima media thickness and relation to ApoE alleles. Atherosclerosis. 2010;**208**:177-182

[36] Slimani A, Harira Y, Trabelsi I, Jomaa W, Maatouk F, Hamda KB, et al. Effect of E670G polymorphism in PCSK9 gene on the risk and severity of coronary heart disease and ischemic stroke in a Tunisian cohort. Journal of Molecular Neuroscience. 2014;**53**:150-157

[37] Chan DC, Pang J, McQuillan BM, Hung J, Beilby JP, Barrett PH, et al. Plasma proprotein convertase subtilisin Kexin type 9 as a predictor of carotid atherosclerosis in asymptomatic adults. Heart, Lung & Circulation. 2016;**25**:520-525

[38] Drouin-Chartier JP, Tremblay AJ, Hogue JC, Ooi TC, Lamarche B, Couture P. The contribution of PCSK9 levels to the phenotypic severity of familial hypercholesterolemia is independent of LDL receptor genotype. Metabolism. 2015;**64**:1541-1547

[39] Alves AC, Etxebarria A, Medeiros AM, Benito-Vicente A, Thedrez A, Passard M, et al. Characterization of the first PCSK9 gain of function homozygote. Journal of the American College of Cardiology. 2015;**66**:2152-2154

[40] Cohen J, Pertsemlidis A, Kotowski IK, Graham R, Garcia CK, Hobbs HH. Low LDL cholesterol in individuals of African descent resulting

from frequent nonsense mutations in PCSK9. Nature Genetics. 2005;**37**:161-165

[41] Hooper AJ, Marais AD, Tanyanyiwa DM, Burnett JR. The C679X mutation in PCSK9 is present and lowers blood cholesterol in a Southern African population. Atherosclerosis. 2007;**193**:445-448

[42] Tsai CW, North KE, Tin A, Haack K, Franceschini N, Saroja Voruganti V, et al. Both rare and common variants in PCSK9 influence plasma low-density lipoprotein cholesterol level in American Indians. The Journal of Clinical Endocrinology and Metabolism. 2015;**100**:E345-E349

[43] Zhao Z, Tuakli-Wosornu Y, Lagace TA, Kinch L, Grishin NV, Horton JD, et al. Molecular characterization of loss-of-function mutations in PCSK9 and identification of a compound heterozygote. American Journal of Human Genetics. 2006;**79**:514-523

[44] Talmud PJ, Shah S, Whittall R, et al. Use of low-density lipoprotein cholesterol gene score to distinguish patients with polygenic and monogenic familial hypercholesterolaemia: A case–control study. Lancet. 2013;**381**:1293-1301

[45] Futema M, Shah S, Cooper JA, et al. Refinement of variant selection for the LDL cholesterol genetic risk score in the diagnosis of the polygenic form of clinical familial hypercholesterolemia and replication in samples from 6 countries. Clinical Chemistry. 2015;**61**:231-238

[46] Wang J, Dron JS, Ban MR, et al. Polygenic versus monogenic causes of hypercholesterolemia ascertained clinically highlights. Arteriosclerosis, Thrombosis, and Vascular Biology. 2016;**36**:2439-2445

[47] Natarajan P, Peloso GM, Zekavat SM, et al. Deep-coverage whole genome sequences and blood lipids among 16,324 individuals. Nature Communications. 2018;**9**:1-12

[48] Esse R, Barroso M, Tavares de Almeida I, Castro R. The contribution of homocysteine metabolism disruption to endothelial dysfunction: State-of-the-art. International Journal of Molecular Sciences. 2019;**20**(4):867

[49] Rosenblatt DS, Lue-Shing H, Arzoumanian A, Low-Nang L, Matiaszuk N. Methylenetetrahydrofolate reductase (MR) deficiency: Thermolability of residual MR activity, methionine synthase activity, and methylcobalamin levels in cultured fibroblasts. Biochemical Medicine and Metabolic Biology. 1992;**47**:221-225

[50] Hankey GJ, Eikelboom JW. Homocysteine and vascular disease. Lancet. 1999;**354**:407-413

[51] Cascella M, Arcamone M, Morelli E, Viscardi D, Russo V, De Franciscis S, et al. Erratum to: Multidisciplinary approach and anesthetic management of a surgical cancer patient with methylene tetrahydrofolate reductase deficiency: A case report and review of the literature. Journal of Medical Case Reports. 2015;**9**:218

[52] Veeranki S, Tyagi SC. Defective homocysteine metabolism: Potential implications for skeletal muscle malfunction. International Journal of Molecular Sciences. 2013;**14**:15074-15091

[53] Hamelet J, Demuth K, Paul JL, Delabar JM, Janel N. Hyperhomocysteinemia due to cystathionine beta synthase deficiency induces dysregulation of genes involved in hepatic lipid homeostasis in mice. Journal of Hepatology. 2007;**46**:151-159

[54] Brustolin S, Giugliani R, Félix TM. Genetics of homocysteine metabolism and associated disorders. Brazilian Journal of Medical and Biological Research. 2010;**43**:1-7

[55] Iqbal MP, Lindblad BS, Mehboobali N, Yusuf FA, Khan AH, Iqbal SP. Folic acid and vitamin B6 deficiencies related hyperhomocysteinemia in apparently healthy Pakistani adults; is mass micronutrient supplementation indicated in this population? Journal of the College of Physicians and Surgeons–Pakistan. 2009;**19**:308-312

[56] Verhoef P, van Vliet T, Olthof MR, Katan MB. A high-protein diet increases postprandial but not fasting plasma total homocysteine concentrations: A dietary controlled, crossover trial in healthy volunteers. The American Journal of Clinical Nutrition. 2005;**82**:553-558

[57] Kamat PK, Mallonee CJ, George AK, Tyagi SC, Tyagi N. Homocysteine, alcoholism, and its potential epigenetic mechanism. Alcoholism, Clinical and Experimental Research. 2016;**40**:2474-2481

[58] Wu CY, Yang M, Lin M, Li LP, Wen XZ. MTHFR C677T polymorphism was an ethnicity-dependent risk factor for cervical cancer development: Evidence based on a meta-analysis. Archives of Gynecology and Obstetrics. 2013;**288**:595-605

[59] Wu YL, Ding XX, Sun YH, Yang HY, Sun L. Methylenetetrahydrofolate reductase (MTHFR) C677T/A1298C polymorphisms and susceptibility to Parkinson's disease: A meta-analysis. Journal of the Neurological Sciences. 2013;**335**:14-21

[60] Undas A, Chojnowski K, Klukowska A, Łętowska M, Mital A, Młynarski W, et al. Determination and interpretation of MTHFR gene mutations in gynecology and internal medicine. Polish Archives of Internal Medicine. 2019;**129**(10):728-732

[61] Jakubowski H. Homocysteine is a protein amino acid in humans: Implications for homocysteine-linked disease. The Journal of Biological Chemistry. 2002;**277**:30425-30428

[62] 136.Jakubowski H. Protein N-homocysteinylation: Implications for atherosclerosis. Biomedicine & Pharmacotherapy. 2001;**55**:443-447

[63] Leiper J, Vallance P. Biological significance of endogenous methylarginines that inhibit nitric oxide synthases. Cardiovascular Research. 1999;**43**:542-548. DOI: 10.1016/S0008-6363(99)00162-5

[64] Miyazaki H, Matsuoka H, Cooke JP, Usui M, Ueda S, Okuda S, et al. Endogenous nitric oxide synthase inhibitor: A novel marker of atherosclerosis. Circulation. 1999;**99**:1141-1146

[65] Nakayama M, Yasue H, Yoshimura M, Shimasaki Y, Kugiyama K, Ogawa H, et al. T-786–>C mutation in the 5′-flanking region of the endothelial nitric oxide synthase gene is associated with coronary spasm. Circulation. 1999;**99**:2864-2870

[66] Rossi GP, Taddei S, Virdis A, Cavallin M, Ghiadoni L, Favilla S, et al. The T-786C and Glu298Asp polymorphisms of the endothelial nitric oxide gene affect the fore arm blood flow responses of Caucasian hypertensive patients. Journal of the American College of Cardiology. 2003;**41**:938-945

[67] Cattaruzza M, Guzik TJ, Slodowski W, Pelvan A, Becker J,

Halle M, et al. Shear stress in sensitivity of endothelial nitric oxide synthase expression as a genetic risk factor for coronary heart disease. Circulation Research. 2004;**95**:841-847

[68] Marsden PA, Heng HH, Scherer SW, Stewart RJ, Hall AV, Shi XM, et al. Structure and chromosomal localization of the human constitutive endothelial nitric oxide synthase gene. The Journal of Biological Chemistry. 1993;**268**:17478-17488

[69] Persu A, Stoenoiu MS, Messiaen T, et al. Modifier effect of ENOS in autosomal dominant polycystic kidney disease. Human Molecular Genetics. 2002;**11**:229-241

[70] McDonald DM, Alp NJ, Channon KM. Functional comparison of the endothelial nitric oxide synthase Glu298Asp polymorphic variants in human endothelial cells. Pharmacogenetics. 2004;**14**:831-839

[71] Jones LC, Tran CTL, Leiper JM, et al. Common genetic variation in a basal promoter element alters DDAH2 expression in endothelial cells. Biochemical and Biophysical Research Communications. 2003;**310**:836-843

[72] Suarez Y, Fernandez-Hernando C, Yu J, Gerber SA, Harrison KD, Pober JS, et al. Dicer-dependent endothelial microRNAs are necessary for postnatal angiogenesis. Proceedings of the National Academy of Sciences of the United States of America. 2008;**105**:14082-14087

[73] Wronska A, Kurkowska-Jastrzebska I, Santulli G. Application of microRNAs in diagnosis and treatment of cardiovascular disease. Acta Physiologica. 2015;**213**:60-83

[74] Akhtar S, Hartmann P, Karshovska E, Rinderknecht FA, Subramanian P, Gremse F, et al. Endothelial hypoxia-inducible factor-1alpha promotes atherosclerosis and monocyte recruitment by upregulating MicroRNA-19a. Hypertension. 2015;**66**:1220-1226

[75] Liu X, Cheng Y, Yang J, Qin S, Chen X, Tang X, et al. Flank sequences of miR-145/143 and their aberrant expression in vascular disease: Mechanism and therapeutic application. Journal of the American Heart Association. 2013;**2**:e000407

[76] Vasan RS, Larson MG, Aragam J, Wang TJ, Mitchell GF, Kathiresan S, et al. Genome-wide association of echocardiographic dimensions, brachial artery endothelial function and treadmill exercise responses in the Framingham heart study. BMC Medical Genetics. 2007;**8**(Suppl 1):S2. DOI: 10.1186/1471-2350-8-S1-S2

[77] Yoshino S, Cilluffo R, Prasad M, Best PJ, Atkinson EJ, Aoki T, et al. Sex-specific genetic variants are associated with coronary endothelial dysfunction. Journal of the American Heart Association. 2016;**5**(4):e002544. DOI: 10.1161/JAHA.115.002544

[78] Ehret GB, Ferreira T, Chasman DI, Jackson AU, Schmidt EM, Johnson T, et al. The genetics of blood pressure regulation and its target organs from association studies in 415 individuals. Nature Genetics. 2016;**48**:1171-1184

[79] Evangelou E, Warren HR, Mosen-Ansorena D, Mifsud B, Pazoki R, Gao H, et al. Genetic analysis of over 1 million people identifies 535 new loci associated with blood pressure traits. Nature Genetics. 2018;**50**:1412-1425

[80] Congrains A, Kamide K, Oguro R, Yasuda O, Miyata K, Yamamoto E, et al. Genetic variants at the 9p21 locus

contribute to atherosclerosis through modulation of ANRIL and CDKN2A/B. Atherosclerosis. 2012;**220**(2):449-455. DOI: 10.1016/j.atherosclerosis.2011.11.017

[81] Chen L, Qu H, Guo M, Zhang Y, Cui Y, Yang Q, et al. ANRIL and atherosclerosis. Journal of Clinical Pharmacy and Therapeutics. 2020;**45**(2):240-248. DOI: 10.1111/jcpt.13060

[82] Paneni F, Costantino S. Diabetes and cardiovascular disease: Let's push forward with translational research. Cardiovascular Diagnosis and Therapy. 2015;**5**(5):407-411. DOI: 10.3978/j.issn.2223-3652.2015.05.12

Section 2

Novel Pathways of Endothelial Dysfunction

Chapter 4

The Role of Occludin in Vascular Endothelial Protection

Yunhui Du, Yanru Duan and Shihan Zhang

Abstract

Endothelial tight junction proteins play an important role in maintaining the integrity of vascular endothelial structure and physiological function. In recent years, studies have found that alterations in the expression, distribution, and structure of endothelial tight junction proteins may lead to many related vascular diseases and pathologies (such as diabetes, atherosclerosis, neurodegenerative diseases, and hypertension). Therefore, related strategies to prevent and/or tight junction proteins dysfunction may be an important therapeutic target. Occludin, as the most representative one among tight junction proteins, is mainly responsible for sealing intercellular junctions, maintaining cell permeability and the integrity of vascular endothelium. Here, we review the published biological information of occludin. We highlight the relationship between occludin and vascular endothelial injury-related disease. At the same time, we show our current knowledge of how vascular endothelial occludin exerts the protective effect and possible clinical applications in the future.

Keywords: occludin, vascular endothelial cells, protective effect

1. Introduction

The normal vascular endothelium is taken as a gatekeeper of cardiovascular health, whereas abnormality of vascular endothelium is a major contributor to a plethora of cardiovascular ailments, such as atherosclerosis, hypertension, myocardial infarction, coronary artery disease [1]. Therefore, it is important to study the occurrence and development mechanism of vascular endothelial injury. Recent studies have shown that alterations in expression, distribution, and structure of endothelial tight junctions (TJ) may lead to atherosclerosis, neurodegenerative diseases, and pulmonary hypertension, suggesting that TJs play an important role in the vascular endothelium [2].

Occludin, the most representative tight junction proteins, can control the permeability of cells by regulating the connection between cells to play a barrier function. Occludin is involved in the formation of cell polarity *via* forming a fence to prevent cells from spreading to the top and base outer membranes [3]. Meanwhile, occludin can promote cell proliferation and migration [4]. In addition, the expression level of occludin in different vascular beds is positively correlated with the properties of the endothelial barrier of the vascular beds. For example, the permeability of the arterial vascular endothelial barrier is lower than that of the venous vascular endothelial barrier, and the expression of occludin in arterial vascular endothelial is about 18 times higher than that in the venous blood vessels [3], suggesting that occludin is a critical factor of cell permeability and plays an important role in maintaining vascular homeostasis.

Alterations in occludin expression play an important role in vascular endothelial dysfunction. For example, the expression of occludin in retinal vascular endothelial cells of diabetics decreased, resulting in vascular dysfunction such as vascular permeability increased, new vascular formation disorders, and inflammatory response increased, suggesting that the decreased level of occludin may be one of the factors for vascular dysfunction in diabetes [5]. Liu et al. [6] isolated primary mouse retinal endothelial cells for *in vitro* culture and found that occludin S490 phosphorylation is one of the important conditions for retinal endothelial cell tube formation, cell proliferation, and migration. In addition, in the rat with cerebral ischemia at 24 h and 72 h, the expression of occludin in the blood-brain barrier first increased and then decreased [7]. In view of this, understanding the role and mechanism of occludin in vascular endothelial protection is significant for the prevention, diagnosis, and treatment of cardiovascular diseases. We will summarize recent advances in the relationship between occludin and vascular endothelial injury based on the biological information of occludin, the signaling pathway of occludin to protect the vascular endothelium, and the relationship between occludin and vascular endothelial injury-related diseases in this chapter.

2. Biological information of occludin

There are four main types of intercellular connections in vertebrates: tight junctions, adhesion junctions, gap junctions, and desmosome junctions. Intercellular tight junctions, which can seal intercellular spaces, control hydronium, water, and other molecular pathways, and maintain cell polarity, as discovered by Farquhar and Palade [8]. Discovery of tight junctions revealed the complexity of cellular internal structural, and cellular tight junction proteins (cingulin [9], Zos [10], Tricellulin, JAM [10], and occludin [11]) further clarify the structural complexity and functional diversity of cells.

2.1 Structure of occludin

Occludin has four transmembrane segments, two extracellular loops (the first extracellular loop rich in tyrosine and glycine and the second extracellular loop rich in tyrosine) and two extracellular loops internal domains (NH2-terminal cytoplasmic domain and COOH-terminal cytoplasmic domain) (**Figure 1**). The main function of the COOH-terminal cytoplasmic domain of occludin is to mediate the basolateral transport and endocytosis of proteins, while occludin lacking the C-terminus can localize at tight junctions, the tight junctions cannot be assembled correctly and function is lost [12]. In addition, Bamforth et al. [13] found that occludin lacking or truncating the N-terminus of the extracellular domain can still target tight junctions and co-localize with ZO-1, but the function of tight junction barrier disappears, suggesting that the C- and N-terminal domains of occludin are involved in tight junction assembly and play a barrier function. In addition, the two extracellular loop domains of occludin are critical for the localization of cellular tight

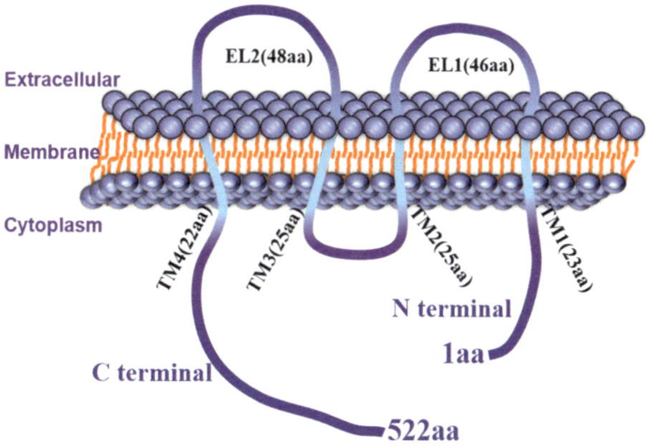

Figure 1.
Structural insight into occludin. Occludin shares with general architecture as tetraspan transmembrane proteins colored in a gradient ranging from yellow at the N-terminus [N] to yellow at the C-terminus [C]. aa: Amino acid; G: Glycine; T: Tyrosine; EL1/2, extracellular loops 1 and 2; TM1 to 4, transmembrane domains 1 to 4.

junctions. Occludin lacking the two extracellular loops is only present on the surface of basal cells but not cellular TJ [14].

2.2 Tissue distribution and expression regulation of occludin

Occludin is expressed in different cells and tissues with different expression level, and it is related to the function of tissues and organs. Occludin can be expressed in human, rat, mouse and other species, and it is mainly localized in arterial and venous vascular endothelial cells, blood-brain barrier, and blood-retinal barrier [14]. Although the expression of occludin could not be detected at the capillary-endothelial junction in mouse heart and skeletal muscle, occludin was highly expressed in brain capillaries [3], suggesting that occludin is essential for regulating the endothelial permeability of the blood-brain barrier. Morcos et al. [15] confirmed that under physiological conditions, occludin is highly expressed in retinal capillaries. However, in pathological conditions, the expression of occludin in the vascular endothelium will decrease significantly accompanied by different stress responses (inflammation, diabetes, cardiovascular diseases, neurodegenerative diseases, and atherosclerosis), and the permeability of vascular endothelium and the apoptosis of cell will increase [4], which suggests that occludin plays an important role in the blood-retinal barrier. In conclusion, under physiological and pathological conditions, the different expression levels of occludin in different tissues and cells are closely related to the tissue barrier properties.

3. The signaling pathway of occludin exerting the protective effect of vascular endothelium

In recent years, the study of cellular tight junction proteins has increased dramatically. Occludin, the most typical cell tight junction protein, has attracted much attention. A large number of studies have shown that many classical signaling pathways are involved in the regulation of occludin, affecting the distribution and expression of occludin.

3.1 Occludin and mTOR pathway

mTOR, consisting of two distinct complexes (mTORC1 and mTORC2), is a sensor of ATP. mTOR1, a classical metabolic pathway in mammals, is involved in the proliferation and migration of vascular endothelial cells [16] and the occurrence and development of various cardiovascular diseases. Currently, a large number of studies have focused on the role of the mTOR pathway in the regulation of occludin expression [1]. In diabetic rat model, as the phosphorylation level of mTOR increases, the downstream 4EBP1 and S6K1 proteins are activated, and the expression level of ROS is increased, which leads to the reduction of NO production in vascular endothelial cells and the decrease of the expression of occludin protein, and the vascular endothelium is damaged. However, the expression of occludin increased after adding the mTOR inhibitor rapamycin [2, 17] inhibiting the production of occludin *via* the inhibition of the PI3K/Akt/mTOR signaling pathway in the cerebral vascular endothelium may lead to the age-related leakage of the blood-brain barrier [3, 18]. Hepatocyte growth factor [HGF] secreted by mesenchymal stromal cells can activate endothelial cell mTOR/STAT3 signaling pathway to promote endothelial occludin expression, maintaining vascular endothelial permeability homeostasis and reducing endothelial cell apoptosis [19]. In conclusion, mTOR signaling pathway is involved in the regulation of occludin expression.

3.2 Occludin and VEGF pathway

The VEGF family consists of five vascular growth factors: VEGFA, VEGFB, VEGFC, VEGFD, and placental growth factor (PIGF). VEGF binds to tyrosine kinase cell receptors (VEGFR1/fms-like tyrosine kinase 1(FLT1), VEGFR2/human kinase insertion domain receptor (KDR)/mouse fetal liver kinase 1 (FLK1), and VEGFR3/fms-like tyrosine kinase 4 (FLT4)) to exert biological effects. Under physiological conditions, VEGF may cause neovascularization, and aggravate vascular inflammation, vascular endothelial cell proliferation, migration and invasion, and endothelial cell survival [20]. A variety of studies revealed the relationship between the VEGF pathway and occludin: (1) Phosphorylation of occludin S490 could induce endothelial cell VEGF expression and promote endothelial cell proliferation and angiogenesis both *in vivo* and *in vitro* [6]; (2) in rat model of cerebral artery occlusion, the lack of VEGF expression in microvascular endothelial cells can prevent the expression of occluding *via* inhibiting the VEGFR2/eNOS signaling pathway to further affect the permeability of the blood-brain barrier [21]; and (3) in mouse mammary cancer model, VEGF secreted by cancer cells can inhibit the expression of occludin in pulmonary vascular endothelium, increase pulmonary vascular permeability, and induce cancer cell metastasis, while overexpression of occludin can alleviate vascular endothelial disorder [22]. In conclusion, the interaction between VEGF and occluding could affect the occurrence and development of the disease.

3.3 Occludin and PKC pathway

PKC, a second messenger-regulated serine/threonine kinase, belongs to the AGA kinase family. Studies have shown that PKC can participate in the regulation of vascular endothelial integrity by interacting with the vascular endothelial marker tight junction protein [23]. Presently, a variety of *in vivo* and *in vitro* disease models have been studied to explore the role of the PKC pathway in regulating the expression and distribution of occludin: (1) In diabetes, metformin improves TJ barrier function by promoting the abundance and assembly of full length occludin at the TJ and that this process involves phosphorylation of the protein *via* an AMPK-PKCζ pathway [24]; (2) high glucose/ethanol induction increases the activity of NAD(P)H and promotes the phosphorylation level of subunit p47phox *via* inhibiting the activity of PKCα and PKCβ to increase the activity of matrix metalloproteinase 2 and reduce the expression of occluding, ultimately increasing vascular endothelial permeability, leading to the loss of blood-brain barrier integrity [25]; (3) in rat model of hypoxia and pulmonary ischemia-reperfusion injury, PKCα inhibits the expression of occludin in cerebral blood vessels and affects cerebral angiogenesis [26]; and (4) endothelial monocyte-activating polypeptide-II (endothelial monocyte-activating polypeptide II, EMAP-II) induced-redistribution of occludin by activating the PKCζ/PP2A signaling pathway is another mechanism in the impairment of the blood-tumor barrier [27].

3.4 Occludin and PKA pathway

PKA, a cAMP-dependent kinase involved in the regulation of vascular endothelium, belongs to AGA kinase. Recently, it was reported in the literature that a novel β-adrenergic receptor agonist [complex 49b]-treated diabetic retinal endothelial cells could activate the PKA signaling pathway, promote the expression of occludin in retinal vascular endothelium, increase vascular tight junctions, and reduce endothelial cell apoptosis [27]. cAMP/PKA signal transduction is involved in the increase of blood-tumor barrier permeability mediated by bradykinin and promotes the up-regulation of occludin expression [28]. Glucagon-like peptide-1 (GLP-1) activates the cAMP/PKA signaling pathway to promote occludin expression and maintain the integrity of the blood-brain barrier in rat primary brain capillary endothelial cells [29].

3.5 Occludin and AMP-activated protein kinase [AMPK] pathway

AMPK is a serine/threonine protein kinase involved in the regulation of cellular and body metabolism. AMPK activation counteracts oxidative stress by inhibiting the production of reactive oxygen derived by NAD[P]H oxidase in endothelial cells [30]. Stimulation of lipopolysaccharide in aging mice can significantly inhibit the activation of AMPK pathway in cerebral vascular endothelial cells, up-regulate the production of NAD[P]H oxidase, and reduce the expression of occludin protein, leading to blood-brain barrier disorders [31]. AMPK kinase inhibits the activation of inflammasome NLRP3 through the mTOR/ULK1 pathway-mediated autophagy, promotes the expression of occludin, and protects the blood-brain barrier in human brain capillary endothelial cells cultured *in vitro* [18]. Studies reported that occludin can negatively regulate AMPK activity to affect blood glucose uptake and energy production [32]. In conclusion, there is a strong connection between the energy metabolism pathway AMPK and occludin.

3.6 Occludin and MAPKs pathway

MAPKs including extracellular signal-related kinases (ERK1/2), p38, and c-Jun N-terminal kinase [JNK] are a family of serine/threonine protein kinases [33]. Under the stimulation of various extracellular factors (such as inflammatory signals), MAPK kinase promotes the activation of nuclear proteins and transcription factors, and regulates gene expression, differentiation, apoptosis and other processes. MAPK kinase is an important intracellular signal transduction that regulates various intracellular functions. Many studies have found that MAPK pathway activation can affect endothelial cell occludin expression and modification in physiological and pathological conditions: (1) Exposure of cerebral microvascular endothelial cells to lipopolysaccharide can affect the p38MAPK/JNK signaling pathway and MMP2 expression, thereby regulating the level of occludin protein in endothelial cells and leading to central nervous system inflammation and brain edema [34]; (2) ERK1/2 inhibits the activation of the NF-κB signaling pathway resulting in the increase of occludin and decrease of endothelial barrier permeability to protect the TJ barrier in human lung microvascular endothelial cells [35]; (3) after lipopolysaccharide stimulates human umbilical vein endothelial cells, it can promote the mRNA and protein expression of CXCL4 and its receptor CXCR3 activates the downstream p38 signaling pathway, thereby inhibiting the expression of occludin in endothelial cells, promoting endothelial cell apoptosis, and increasing endothelial cell permeability [36]; (4) exposure of human umbilical vein endothelial cells to γ-rays can promote the expression of MAPK pathway molecules p38, p53, p21, and p27, induce the activation of NF-κB signaling pathway, and inhibit the expression of occludin in endothelial cells, resulting in the increase of cell permeability, oxidative stress, nitrification, and inflammatory [37]; (5) in human brain microvascular endothelial cells, reduction of occludin can upregulate PI3K/AKT and ERK signaling pathways, and promote cytokine secretion, inflammatory factor activation, and apoptosis protein expression. However, overexpression of occludin can inhibit endothelial cell apoptosis and inflammation [25]. In conclusion, the MAPK signaling pathway is closely related to the regulation of occludin.

4. Protein post-translational modifications (PTMs)

In general, various protein post-translational modifications (PTMs) increase the functional diversity of the proteome through adding covalent functional groups, proteolytically cleaving regulatory subunits, or degrading the entire protein. These covalent modifications of proteins involving in phosphorylation, glycosylation, ubiquitination, nitrosylation, methylation, acetylation, lipidation, and proteolysis have affected all the details of cellular physiology and pathology. The post-translational modifications of proteins further contribute to the biological complexity from genome to proteome. PTMs play an important role in regulating activity, localization, and interaction with cellular molecules (such as proteins, nucleic acids, lipids, and cofactors) [38, 39].

Therefore, better understanding and analysis of protein post-translational modifications may be crucial for the study of cell biology, disease treatment and disease prevention including cardiovascular diseases, several forms of cancers, neurodegenerative diseases and diabetes, etc. [40].

4.1 Post-translational modifications of occludin

In recent years, post-translational modifications of occludin, as representative tight junction proteins, have become a research hotspot. The reported post-translational modifications of occludin include proteolysis, phosphorylation, and ubiquitination, which have all been shown to play vital roles in the course of disease occurrence, development, and convalescence [41, 42].

4.2 Proteolytic degradation of occludin

Studies have found that degradation of tight junction proteins play an important regulatory feature in pathological and physiological tissue remodeling [43]. Basic studies demonstrated that the two fragments of cleaved Occludin released into circulation and the levels of blood occludin correlate well with the extent of blood brain barrier in cerebral ischemic model of rats [44]. In addition, occludin serve as a potential biomarker to predict the severity of acute ischemic stroke, hemorrhagic transformation, and patient prognosis [45]. These results suggested that the degradation of Occludin may be involved in the occurrence and development of many diseases.

4.3 MMPs-dependent degradation of occludin

Matrix metalloproteinases (MMPs) are secreted by astrocytes, endothelial cells, pericytes and peripheral circulating cells and are capable to degrade extracellular matrix (ECM) proteins as well as non-ECM proteins, including cytokines, chemokines, membrane receptors, and antimicrobial peptides [46, 47]. Studied showed that MMPs are related to the development of cancer infiltration and metastasis, inflammatory response, and angiogenesis. Within the endothelial layer, MMPs can degrade intercellular junction molecules (such as cadherin, occludin, and claudins) and intracellular structural proteins (e.g., actins), enhancing the permeability of endothelial barrier [48].

Currently, a number of data have showed that occludin was mainly proteolytically cleaved *via* MMPs to inactive fragments, leading to endothelial barrier disruption. (1) Feng Chen et al. demonstrated MMP9 induced the degradation of occludin and suppressed the synthesis and expression of Occludin in brain endothelial cells and in brains of mice with experimental acute liver failure (ALF), which can cause severe vasogenic brain edema [49]. (2) Related studies showed that LPS/hypoxia induced brain blood barrier (BBB) leakage by MMP2/MMP9 contributed to the degradation of occludin in brain microvascular endothelial cells [34]. (3) TGF-β can promote the production of MMP9 in brain microvascular endothelial cells and retinal endothelial cells, accelerate the degradation of Occludin, and lead to increased vascular endothelial permeability [50]. (4) Several studies demonstrated that MMP2/9 leads to occludin fragmentation in brain microvessels from rat model of cerebral ischemic injury, with resultant brain leakage and brain edema [51–53]. (5) At the same time, Yang et al. firstly described the temporal dynamics of occludin degradation by MMPs in rodent models of cerebral ischemic injury, suggesting that MMP-2 cleaved occludin during the early phase of the ischemia (3 h), while MMP-9 caused further occludin degradation and more long-term (24-h) alterations to BBB integrity. In addition, MMP9 can promote the degradation of occludin through HIF-1α and AQP-4, ultimately triggering BBB disruption and brain edema [54]. (6) Simultaneous data show that MMP2/9-mediated occludin hydrolysis can be used as a marker of blood-brain barrier and blood-retinal barrier in type 2 diabetes and diabetic retinopathy [55, 56]. (7) Caron et al. have suggested that elevated ProMMP-2/9 and MMP9 correlate with increased levels of occludin degradation in rodent kidney endothelium in ischemic injury [57]. (8) The degradation of tight junction proteins (occludin, claudins) through MMP9 secreted by glioma cells is an important mechanism in the BBB breakdown mediated by TGF-β [58]. (9) In acute leukemia, MMP9 secreted by leukemic cells degraded occludin, which constituted an extreme mechanism of the BBB breakdown that contributes to the invasion of the central nervous system [59]. Overall, occludin contains extracellular MMP cleavage sites and are a substrate of MMPs. In endothelial cells, the degradation of Occludin mediated by MMPs leads to vascular leakage.

4.4 MMP-independent proteolysis of occludin

At present, a large number of data focus on MMPs-dependent occludin degradation; however, there are also some studies showing the existence of MMPs-independent occludin degradation. (1) Qian et al. found that tryptase can act on mouse brain microvascular endothelial cells to promote the production of MMP9/2, degrade the tight junction proteins occludin and Claudin5, and lead to the destruction of the blood-brain barrier [60]. (2) Wan et al. and Runs et al. verified both serine and cysteine peptidases cleavage the occludin with elevation of epithelial permeability, which reveals a pathological mechanism for allergen delivery across lung and nasal epithelial barriers in asthma and allergic rhinitis sufferers [35]. (3) Caspase-mediated cleavage of the occludin C-terminal promotes apoptosis in MDCKs [61]. The studies about the MMP-independent proteolysis of occludin occurred in the epithelial cells; therefore, more research is needed to further define the MMP-independent proteolysis of occludin in endothelial cells.

4.5 Occludin phosphorylation

Protein phosphorylation is a ubiquitous type of post-translational modification, whereby protein kinase catalyzes the phosphorylation reactions by transferring the phosphate group of ATP to the substrate protein amino acid residues, typically serine, threonine, and tyrosine, or bind GTP under the action of signal transduction. It was widely demonstrated that protein phosphorylation is the most basic and the most common key mechanism for regulating and controlling protein biological activity and function [62]. Notably, the phosphorylation status of occludin regulating endothelial barrier protection has been received extensive attention.

More than 40 phosphorylation residues are in human occludin; however, only nine sites are confirmed in cell levels by different kinases on certain stimuli, including Y398, T400, Y402, T403, T404, S408, T424, T438, and S490 [46]. All confirmed phosphorylation residues lie in the occludin C terminal. As early as 1997, Sakakibara et al. firstly observed increased phospho-serine [pSer] and phospho-threonine [pThr] occludin selectively localized to intact epithelial TJs as a detergent-insoluble form [63]. Subsequently, Kale and Elias et al. confirmed occludin phosphorylation on key serine, threonine, and tyrosine residues plays a crucial role in the assembly and maintenance of TJs in Caco-2 and MDCK cells [64, 65]. Dörfel and colleagues in 2013 studied that CK2-mediated phosphorylation [T400A/T404A/S408A] of occludin in MDCK-C11 cells bind with ZO1/2 interaction and protect the epithelial barrier [66]. The regulation of occludin phosphorylation in endothelium has also received extensive attention, with many studies focusing on how the phosphorylation status of occludin regulates the vessel barrier.

Different phosphorylation sites of occludin exerts specific functions in endothelial cells: (1) Antonetti and his colleagues investigate the role of tight junction protein occludin phosphorylation at S490 in modulating barrier properties and its impact on visual function. They found that endothelial-specific expression of the S490A form of occludin completely prevented diabetes-induced permeability to label dextran and inhibit leukostasis. Importantly, vascular-specific expression of the occludin mutant completely blocked the diabetes-induced decrease in visual acuity and contrast sensitivity in the retinas of streptozotocin-induced diabetic mice [67]. (2) Treatment with glutamate increased tyrosine phosphorylation and decreased threonine phosphorylation of occluding in brain microvascular endothelial cells. It affects the redistribution of occludin. These may lead to opening of the blood-brain barrier (BBB) and induce further brain damage [68]. (3) The phosphorylation of occludin and claudin-5 by RhoK at specific sites disrupted the integrity of BBB. Antibodies against specific phosphorylation sites of occludin could be useful reagents for monitoring BBB dysfunction *in vivo* [69]. (4) Other recent studies confirm the importance of threonine phosphorylation with occludin C-terminal for mediating its ability to localize to the tight junction [70–72]. According to the above studies, it is demonstrated that the specific phosphorylation sites of occludin regulate the different function of endothelial cells. Other studies need to further focus on other phosphorylation residues of occludin in correlating with endothelial function.

4.6 Occludin ubiquitination

Ubiquitination, also known as ubiquitylation, refers to the process in which the ubiquitin (a small 76-residue regulatory protein widely expressed in eukaryotes) molecules classify the proteins in cells under the action of a series of special enzymes, choose the target protein molecules from them, and specifically modify the target proteins. These special enzymes include ubiquitin-activating enzymes (E1), ubiquitin-conjugating enzymes (E2), ubiquitin-protein ligase (E3), and degrading enzymes [73]. Ubiquitination plays an important role in protein localization, metabolism, function, regulation, and degradation [73, 74]. At the same time, ubiquitination takes part within the regulation of nearly all life activities, including cell cycle, proliferation, apoptosis, differentiation, metastasis, gene expression, transcriptional regulation, signal transmission, damage repair, inflammation, and immunity [73, 74]. In recent years, studies about the functional role of occludin ubiquitination in diseases have begun to emerge in a burst. And the modification way has become an important regulatory mechanism in epithelial and endothelial function.

Hannelore et al. identified a novel interaction between occludin N-terminal and the E3 ubiquitin-protein ligase Itch, a member of the HECT domain-containing ubiquitin-protein ligases by co-immunoprecipitation *in vivo* and *in vitro* [75]. In addition, the team provides evidence that Itch is specifically involved in the ubiquitination of occludin *in vivo*, and that the degradation of occludin is sensitive to proteasome inhibition. The team firstly confirmed that occludin can be ubiquitinated. Liu and Lee et al. reported that occludin degradation was associated with Itch and UBC-4 (an ubiquitin-conjugating enzyme), resulting in occludin ubiquitination to disrupt tight junctions in blood and testosterone barrier [76]. A slightly later study reported that a conserved C-terminal PY motif of occludin association with Nedd4-2 was involved in the paracellular permeability of mpk-CCD[c14] cells (a collecting duct epithelial cell line) by coimmunoprecipitation. These authors also showed that small interfering RNA [siRNA]-mediated knockdown of Nedd4-2 increased occludin expression and reduced the epithelial permeability, with Nedd4-2 overexpression having the opposite effects [77]. In conclusion, ubiquitinated occludin is taken part in the maintenance of cell barrier.

Currently, the study about the regulation of occludin ubiquitination in vascular endothelial function focuses on the following aspects. (1) Murakami et al. demonstrated that Ser-490 phosphorylation of occludin is an essential prerequisite for its ubiquitination in BRECs. The team showed that a C-terminal occludin-ubiquitin chimera was internalized, bypassing the requirement for phosphorylation. Thus, VEGF, through PKCβ-mediated phosphorylation, promotes Itch-mediated ubiquitylation of occludin, which is required for its internalization and degradation, thereby enhancing retinal endothelial permeability [78]. (2) It is well known that blood-spinal cord barrier (BSCB) breakdown is a hallmark of amyotrophic lateral sclerosis (ALS). Results found that mutant SOD1 induced occludin phosphorylation, which promoted the subsequent occludin ubiquitination mediated by the E3 ligase ITCH. Moreover, ubiquitinated occludin interacted with Eps15 to initiate its internalization, then trafficked to Rab5-positive vesicles, and be degraded by proteasomes, resulting in a reduction in cell surface localization and total abundance [79]. (3) Feng et al. showed that the γ-secretase blocker DAPT reduced the permeability of the BBB by decreasing the ubiquitination and degradation of occludin during permanent brain ischemia [80]. Notwithstanding the information already generated about the role of occludin ubiquitination in endothelial cells, several avenues for future investigation still remain. The identification of new ubiquitin enzymes, characterization of tissue and cell-specific occludin ubiquitination, and deciphering the functional rapport between different modification events (e.g., phosphorylation, ubiquitination, proteolysis), will likely typify future studies in this field. This will ultimately yield a fuller understanding of how ubiquitination modifications to occludin affect TJ characteristics and will help to unlock the therapeutic potential of the TJ by identifying new cellular targets for intervention in diseases characterized by barrier dysregulation.

5. The relationship between occludin and vascular endothelial injury-related diseases

Vascular endothelial injury includes vasodilation dysfunction characterized by decreased endothelial NO and structural damage characterized by increased endothelial inflammatory response, endothelial cell apoptosis, and endothelial cell permeability. A large number of studies have found that the abnormal expression and modification of occludin is accompanied by damage to the endothelial structure of blood vessels in tissues and organs, resulting in increased vascular permeability, inflammatory cell infiltration, and apoptosis. Therefore, we will detail the relationship between occludin and diseases related to damage to the arterial vascular endothelial structure in this section.

5.1 Occludin and arterial vascular disease

5.1.1 Occludin and cerebrovascular injury-related diseases

Brain has received extensive attention because it is the most vulnerable to endothelial barrier dysfunction. Under normal circumstances, the blood-brain barrier is a semi-permeable interface, which is important for providing a neuronal microenvironment and exchanging water, ions, gases, and metabolites, but it is not suitable for exogenous harmful substances such as bacteria and viruses [4]. However, many triggers (e.g., inflammation, traumatic brain injury, ischemia) can lead to leakage of the blood-brain barrier, increasing the risk of cerebral edema, nerve damage, cerebral hemorrhage, and further increasing the risk of cerebral ischemia. The brain endothelial cell tight junction protein occludin plays an important role in maintaining the integrity of the blood-brain barrier. For example: (1) Both clinical and basic researchers have found that under cerebral ischemia, and cysteinase can hydrolyze the blood-brain barrier tight junction protein occludin to promote its release into the blood, resulting in an increase of occludin levels in serum. Therefore, serum occludin levels can be used as an indicator for predicting the severity of acute ischemic stroke, hemorrhagic transformation, and prognosis of patients [45]; (2) studies have shown that the increased permeability of the blood-brain barrier in type 1 diabetic mice may be due to the increased level of serum extracellular vesicle occludin, which affects the distribution of occludin in the cerebral vascular endothelial cell membrane [81]; (3) in rat model of traumatic shock, the expression of occludin in cerebral vascular endothelial cells is reduced, which affects the integrity of the blood-brain barrier, the leakage of inflammatory cells, and deterioration of vascular inflammatory response [82]; (4) both *in vitro* and *in vivo* studies found that the occludin degradation caused by autophagy is an important factor of the blood-brain barrier disorder when the brain is exposed to an ischemic environment [83]; (5) the increased expression of occludin in cerebral microvascular endothelial cells can reduce the apoptosis of endothelial cells by inhibiting the expression of apoptosis-related proteins, and the degradation of occludin makes cerebral blood vessels more prone to reperfusion injury [25, 84]; (6) in diabetic animal model, the expression of occludin in the cerebral vascular endothelium is reduced, which is manifested as diabetes complicated with cerebrovascular disease, and nerve damage, etc. [85]. In conclusion, abnormal expression, modification, and degradation of occludin may induce vascular endothelial dysfunction, resulting in injury of blood-brain barrier function, and ultimately aggravating the occurrence and development of brain diseases.

5.1.2 Occludin and coronary vascular injury diseases

Coronary endothelial barrier dysfunction is closely related to ischemic heart disease. Endothelial barrier integrity and function are regulated by a variety of transmembrane proteins, including claudin family proteins, occludin, VE-cadherin, etc. In recent years, basic research on occludin and coronary artery injury-related diseases has found that in mouse model of coronary artery sclerosis, the expression of occludin in arterial endothelial cells decreased, and the atherosclerotic plaque was expanded. Conversely, up-regulation of occludin expression in arterial endothelial cells can alleviate the occurrence and development of plaque [86]. In conclusion, abnormal expression of occludin in coronary endothelial cells is directly related to the occurrence and development of heart disease.

5.1.3 Occludin and pulmonary vascular injury diseases

Pulmonary vascular endothelial cells form a complete cell barrier, participate in the regulation of vascular homeostasis, and maintain the normal operation of the body. Under pathological conditions (diabetes, hypertension, and hyperlipidemia), the pulmonary vascular endothelial barrier is damaged, resulting in vascular endothelial dysfunction and chronic structural damage. Tight junction proteins play an important role in maintaining the integrity of the pulmonary vascular endothelial barrier. As an important component of TJ, occludin has been shown to be down-regulated in a variety of pulmonary vascular injury-related diseases. (1) Pulmonary arterial hypertension (PAH) is a progressive disease characterized by pulmonary endothelial cell dysfunction and vascular remodeling. Histological evaluation of mouse model of pulmonary arterial hypertension shows downregulation of occludin expression in pulmonary vessels [87]; (2) the expression of occludin in pulmonary artery endothelial cells of diabetic and hypertensive model mice was reduced, and nitric oxide (NO), superoxide dismutase, and inducible NO synthase were severely imbalanced, suggesting that occludin may be involved in the production of vascular endothelial NO [88]; (3) studies have found that the occludin protein in the pulmonary artery endothelial cells of the rat model of acute lung injury is lost, the endothelial permeability is increased, the vascular inflammatory response is increased, and oxidative stress and other pathological states occur [89]. In conclusion, abnormal expression and distribution of occludin are closely related to pulmonary vascular lesions.

5.1.4 Occludin and renal vascular injury diseases

Kidney is one of the organs with the most abundant distribution of endothelial cells. Under physiological conditions, renal endothelium can mediate signal communication between various parts of the kidney, stabilize renal osmotic pressure, and regulate vascular permeability. Under pathological conditions such as ischemia, inflammation, and sepsis, renal vascular endothelial permeability is increased, renal metabolism is impaired, and the basal layer of endothelial cells is thickened, which induces endothelial damage and leads to plasma leakage. Occludin is involved in maintaining the barrier function of renal endothelial cells, and a large number of basic studies on occludin and renal vascular injury have found that (1) The abnormal expression and distribution of occludin in renal endothelial cells, the imbalance of electrolytes such as sodium, potassium, and chloride, and the deterioration of renal injury exist in the rat model of renal ischemia-reperfusion, suggesting that the abnormal expression and distribution of occludin in renal vascular endothelial cells affect renal function homeostasis [90]; (2) High glucose and high fat stimulate human glomerular endothelial cells, decrease the expression of occludin, and damage renal endothelial barrier function, which leads to development of diabetic nephropathy [91]; (3) renal dysfunction caused by hyperoxia is closely related to renal endothelial tight junction protein occludin [92]. In conclusion, the decreased expression of occludin in renal endothelial cells under pathological conditions may be a new marker of renal vascular injury.

5.1.5 Occludin and other arterial diseases

The blood retinal endothelial barrier maintains the integrity of retinal tissue. The level of occludin in endothelial cells can dynamically regulate the intracellular signal transduction system, promote the transport of nutrients, and limit the transport of harmful substances, which is extremely important for maintaining the blood retinal endothelial barrier. Studies have found that: (1) The phosphorylation of occludin S490 in retinal endothelial cells regulates the proliferation and angiogenesis of retinal endothelial cells [6]; (2) the decreased expression of occludin in endothelial cells of diabetic retinopathy can induce inflammatory cell infiltration, suggesting that the loss of occludin at the blood-retinal barrier leads to increased endothelial cell permeability, which is an important factor for mediating the aggravation of vascular inflammatory responses [93]; (3) when neonatal rats exposed to hypoxia, the expression of occludin in retinal endothelial cells decreased, vacuoles appeared in endothelial cytoplasm, and mitochondrial vacuoles and multivesicles accumulated in capillary lumen, suggesting that occludin was involved in the occurrence of hypoxic stress response [94]; (4) relevant studies have shown that exogenous stimuli (high sugar, long-term high-fat diet, long-term smoking) can inhibit the expression of occludin in the vascular endothelium, resulting in an increase in vascular permeability, which in turn causes the occurrence of oxidative stress in vascular endothelial cells [89]. According to the above research results, it is suggested that the maintenance of blood retinal endothelial barrier integrity is closely related to occludin.

5.2 Occludin and venous vascular diseases

Venous vessels maintain venous barrier function by expressing abundant occludin. Recent studies on occludin in venous endothelial cells have shown that: (1) Serum occludin levels are higher in patients with jugular vein stenosis [95]; (2) Nitta et al. found that in mouse model of retinal vein occlusion, venous vascular inflammation increased, occludin expression decreased, and retinal edema occurred; conversely, inhibiting vascular inflammation could alleviate the decrease in occludin expression and maintain retinal homeostasis [96]; (3) studies on mice with ischemic stroke found that early cerebral venous filling and dilation were associated with occludin displacement and abnormal expression and distribution [97]. In conclusion, the maintenance of the venous homeostasis is inseparable from the regulation of occludin.

6. Conclusions

Occludin, as a cellular tight junction protein, mediates molecular communication between cells and maintains the integrity of various tissues and cells. More and more studies have confirmed that under pathological conditions, various signaling pathways can disrupt the integrity of cell barrier by regulating the expression and distribution of occludin, and participate in apoptosis, inflammation, cardiovascular and neurodegenerative diseases. Occludin plays an important role in cardiovascular disease, but current research also faces great challenges. A variety of classical signaling pathways can regulate the expression and distribution of occludin, but only some studies suggest that occludin can act as an upstream regulatory molecule to affect downstream signaling pathways, whether it affects multiple molecules and signaling pathways is an urgent problem to be solved. At present, most researches focus on occludin participating in cell barrier and maintaining cell integrity. Whether its overexpression plays a positive role in all systems is unknown. Loss of occludin can affect vascular endothelial permeability, leading to pathology such as inflammatory cell infiltration, apoptosis, and oxidative stress. However, whether inflammatory stimulation, apoptosis, and oxidative stress can directly affect the expression, modification, and redistribution of occludin is the current vacancy in current research field and needs further exploration and discovery. Relatively speaking, the research on occludin and vascular endothelial injury-related diseases is still very limited, but there is already relevant evidence that it is a close relationship between them. There is still a large gap in the relationship between occludin and vascular metabolic diseases needs to be filled. With further research in the future, the connection between occludin and many diseases related to vascular endothelial injury will become increasingly clear. In a word, whether it is possible to inhibit or use occludin to develop related drugs and apply them to the treatment of clinical diseases requires further research and discovery.

Conflict of interest

The authors declare no conflict of interest.

Author details

Yunhui Du[1]*, Yanru Duan[2] and Shihan Zhang[3]

1 Beijing Institute of Heart, Lung and Blood Vessel Diseases, Beijing Anzhen Hospital, Capital Medical University, Beijing, P.R. China

2 Department of Physiology and Pathophysiology, School of Basic Medical Sciences, Capital Medical University, Beijing, P.R. China

3 Medical Oncology Department, Pediatric Oncology Center, Beijing Children's Hospital, Capital Medical University, National Center for Children's Health, Beijing Key Laboratory of Pediatric Hematology Oncology, Key Laboratory of Major Diseases in Children, Ministry of Education, Beijing, P.R. China

*Address all correspondence to: annahhdu820@mail.ccmu.edu.cn

IntechOpen

© 2022 The Author(s). Licensee IntechOpen. This chapter is distributed under the terms of the Creative Commons Attribution License (http://creativecommons.org/licenses/by/3.0), which permits unrestricted use, distribution, and reproduction in any medium, provided the original work is properly cited.

References

[1] Sun HJ, Wu ZY, Nie XW, Bian JS. Role of endothelial dysfunction in cardiovascular diseases: The link between inflammation and hydrogen sulfide. Frontiers in Pharmacology. 2019;**10**:1568

[2] Li X, Wu TT, Chen J, Qiu W. Elevated expression levels of serum insulin-like growth factor-1, tumor necrosis factor-α and vascular endothelial growth factor 165 might exacerbate type 2 diabetic nephropathy. Journal of Diabetes Investigation. 2017;**8**(1):108-114

[3] Cong X, Kong W. Endothelial tight junctions and their regulatory signaling pathways in vascular homeostasis and disease. Cellular Signalling. 2020;**66**:109485

[4] Keep RF, Andjelkovic AV, Xiang J, Stamatovic SM, Antonetti DA, Hua Y, et al. Brain endothelial cell junctions after cerebral hemorrhage: Changes, mechanisms and therapeutic targets. Journal of Cerebral Blood Flow and Metabolism. 2018;**38**(8):1255-1275

[5] Chen YH, Xu X, Sheng MJ, Zheng Z, Gu Q. Effects of asymmetric dimethylarginine on bovine retinal capillary endothelial cell proliferation, reactive oxygen species production, permeability, intercellular adhesion molecule-1, and occludin expression. Molecular Vision. 2011;**17**:332-340

[6] Liu X, Dreffs A, Díaz-Coránguez M, Runkle EA, Gardner TW, Chiodo VA, et al. Occludin S490 phosphorylation regulates vascular endothelial growth factor-induced retinal neovascularization. The American Journal of Pathology. 2016;**186**(9):2486-2499

[7] Zinnanti WJ, Lazovic J, Housman C, Antonetti DA, Koeller DM, Connor JR, et al. Mechanism of metabolic stroke and spontaneous cerebral hemorrhage in glutaric aciduria type I. Acta Neuropathologica Communications. 2014;**2**:13

[8] Farquhar MG, Palade GE. Junctional complexes in various epithelia. The Journal of Cell Biology. 1963;**17**(2):375-412

[9] Citi S, Sabanay H, Jakes R, Geiger B, Kendrick-Jones J. Cingulin, a new peripheral component of tight junctions. Nature. 1988;**333**(6170):272-276

[10] Itoh M, Nagafuchi A, Yonemura S, Kitani-Yasuda T, Tsukita S, Tsukita S. The 220-kD protein colocalizing with cadherins in non-epithelial cells is identical to ZO-1, a tight junction-associated protein in epithelial cells: cDNA cloning and immunoelectron microscopy. The Journal of Cell Biology. 1993;**121**(3):491-502

[11] Furuse M, Hirase T, Itoh M, Nagafuchi A, Yonemura S, Tsukita S, et al. Occludin: A novel integral membrane protein localizing at tight junctions. The Journal of Cell Biology. 1993;**123**(6 Pt 2):1777-1788

[12] Balda MS, Flores-Maldonado C, Cereijido M, Matter K. Multiple domains of occludin are involved in the regulation of paracellular permeability. Journal of Cellular Biochemistry. 2000;**78**(1):85-96

[13] Bamforth SD, Kniesel U, Wolburg H, Engelhardt B, Risau W. A dominant mutant of occludin disrupts tight junction structure and function. Journal of Cell Science. 1999;**112**(Pt 12):1879-1888

[14] Heinemann U, Schuetz A. Structural features of tight-junction proteins.

International Journal of Molecular Sciences. 2019;**20**(**23**):6020

[15] Morcos Y, Hosie MJ, Bauer HC, Chan-Ling T. Immunolocalization of occludin and claudin-1 to tight junctions in intact CNS vessels of mammalian retina. Journal of Neurocytology. 2001;**30**(2):107-123

[16] Li Y, Xu Q, Shi M, Gan P, Huang Q, Wang A, et al. Low-level laser therapy induces human umbilical vascular endothelial cell proliferation, migration and tube formation through activating the PI3K/Akt signaling pathway. Microvascular Research. 2020;**129**:103959

[17] Wang GH, Ma KL, Zhang Y, Hu ZB, Liu L, Lu J, et al. Platelet microparticles contribute to aortic vascular endothelial injury in diabetes via the mTORC1 pathway. Acta Pharmacologica Sinica. 2019;**40**(4):468-476

[18] Manthari RK, Tikka C, Ommati MM, Niu R, Sun Z, Wang J, et al. Arsenic induces autophagy in developmental mouse cerebral cortex and hippocampus by inhibiting PI3K/Akt/mTOR signaling pathway: Involvement of blood-brain barrier's tight junction proteins. Archives of Toxicology. 2018;**92**(11):3255-3275

[19] Meng SS, Guo FM, Zhang XW, Chang W, Peng F, Qiu HB, et al. mTOR/STAT-3 pathway mediates mesenchymal stem cell-secreted hepatocyte growth factor protective effects against lipopolysaccharide-induced vascular endothelial barrier dysfunction and apoptosis. Journal of Cellular Biochemistry. 2019;**120**(3):3637-3650

[20] Ashina K, Tsubosaka Y, Kobayashi K, Omori K, Murata T. VEGF-induced blood flow increase causes vascular hyper-permeability in vivo. Biochemical and Biophysical Research Communications. 2015;**464**(2):590-595

[21] Wang Q, Deng Y, Huang L, Zeng W, Chen S, Lv B, et al. Hypertonic saline downregulates endothelial cell-derived VEGF expression and reduces blood-brain barrier permeability induced by cerebral ischaemia via the VEGFR2/eNOS pathway. International Journal of Molecular Medicine. 2019;**44**(3):1078-1090

[22] Li R, Qi Y, Jiang M, Zhang T, Wang H, Wang L, et al. Primary tumor-secreted VEGF induces vascular hyperpermeability in premetastatic lung via the occludin phosphorylation/ubiquitination pathway. Molecular Carcinogenesis. 2019;**58**(12):2316-2326

[23] Jo H, Hwang D, Kim JK, Lim YH. Oxyresveratrol improves tight junction integrity through the PKC and MAPK signaling pathways in Caco-2 cells. Food and Chemical Toxicology. 2017;**108**(Pt A):203-213

[24] Kalsi KK, Garnett JP, Patkee W, Weekes A, Dockrell ME, Baker EH, et al. Metformin attenuates the effect of Staphylococcus aureus on airway tight junctions by increasing PKCζ-mediated phosphorylation of occludin. Journal of Cellular and Molecular Medicine. 2019;**23**(1):317-327

[25] Yu H, Wang C, Wang X, Wang H, Zhang C, You J, et al. Long-term exposure to ethanol downregulates tight junction proteins through the protein kinase Cα signaling pathway in human cerebral microvascular endothelial cells. Experimental and Therapeutic Medicine. 2017;**14**(5):4789-4796

[26] Xia W, Pan Z, Zhang H, Zhou Q, Liu Y. Inhibition of ERRα aggravates sepsis-induced acute lung injury in rats via provoking inflammation and

oxidative stress. Oxidative Medicine and Cellular Longevity. 2020;**2020**:2048632

[27] Li Z, Liu YH, Liu XB, Xue YX, Wang P, Liu LB. Low-dose endothelial monocyte-activating polypeptide-II increases permeability of blood-tumor barrier via a PKC-ζ/PP2A-dependent signaling mechanism. Experimental Cell Research. 2015;**331**(2):257-266

[28] Boardman R, Pang V, Malhi N, Lynch AP, Leach L, Benest AV, et al. Activation of notch signaling by soluble Dll4 decreases vascular permeability via a cAMP/PKA-dependent pathway. American Journal of Physiology. Heart and Circulatory Physiology. 2019;**316**(5):H1065-H1075

[29] Yue W, Li Y, Ou D, Yang Q. The GLP-1 receptor agonist liraglutide protects against oxidized LDL-induced endothelial inflammation and dysfunction via KLF2. IUBMB Life. 2019;**71**(9):1347-1354

[30] Xiong R, Zhou XG, Tang Y, Wu JM, Sun YS, Teng JF, et al. Lychee seed polyphenol protects the blood-brain barrier through inhibiting Aβ[25-35]-induced NLRP3 inflammasome activation via the AMPK/mTOR/ULK1-mediated autophagy in bEnd.3 cells and APP/PS1 mice. Phytotherapy Research. 2021;**35**(2):954-973

[31] Wang X, Xue GX, Liu WC, Shu H, Wang M, Sun Y, et al. Melatonin alleviates lipopolysaccharide-compromised integrity of blood-brain barrier through activating AMP-activated protein kinase in old mice. Aging Cell. 2017;**16**(2):414-421

[32] Victor C, Marta S, Jorge L, Jane H, Neil S, Martina V. Occludin regulates glucose uptake and ATP production in pericytes by influencing AMP-activated protein kinase activity. Journal of Cerebral Blood Flow and Metabolism. 2018;**38**(2):317-332

[33] Liu Y, Tang J, Yuan J, Yao C, Hosoi K, Han Y, et al. Arsenite-induced downregulation of occludin in mouse lungs and BEAS-2B cells via the ROS/ERK/ELK1/MLCK and ROS/p38 MAPK signaling pathways. Toxicology Letters. 2020;**332**:146-154

[34] Qin LH, Huang W, Mo XA, Chen YL, Wu XH. LPS induces occludin dysregulation in cerebral microvascular endothelial cells via MAPK signaling and augmenting MMP-2 levels. Oxidative Medicine and Cellular Longevity. 2015;**2015**:120641

[35] Zhou Q, Wang YW, Ni PF, Chen YN, Dong HQ, Qian YN. Effect of tryptase on mouse brain microvascular endothelial cells via protease-activated receptor 2. Journal of Neuroinflammation. 2018;**15**(**1**):248

[36] Wang X, Zhao Z, Zhu K, Bao R, Meng Y, Bian J, et al. Effects of CXCL4/CXCR3 on the lipopolysaccharide-induced injury in human umbilical vein endothelial cells. Journal of Cellular Physiology. 2019;**234**(12):22378-22385

[37] Wang H, Segaran RC, Chan LY, Aladresi AAM, Chinnathambi A, Alharbi SA, et al. Gamma radiation-induced disruption of cellular junctions in HUVECs is mediated through affecting mapk/nf-κb inflammatory pathways. Oxidative Medicine and Cellular Longevity. 2019;**2019**:1486232

[38] Patwardhan A, Cheng N, Trejo J. Post-translational modifications of G protein-coupled receptors control cellular Signaling dynamics in space and time. Pharmacological Reviews. 2021;**73**:120-151

[39] Banks CJ, Andersen JL. Mechanisms of SOD1 regulation by post-translational

modifications. Redox Biology. 2019;**26**:101270

[40] Song L, Luo ZQ. Post-translational regulation of ubiquitin signaling. The Journal of Cell Biology. 2019;**218**:1776-1786

[41] Majolée J, Kovačević I, Hordijk PL. Ubiquitin-based modifications in endothelial cell-cell contact and inflammation. Journal of Cell Science. 2019;**132**:jcs227728

[42] Cummins PM. Occludin: One protein, many forms. Molecular and Cellular Biology. 2012;**32**:242-250

[43] Reiche J, Huber O. Post-translational modifications of tight junction transmembrane proteins and their direct effect on barrier function. Biochimica et biophysica acta. Biomembranes. 2020;**1862**:183330

[44] Pan R, Yu K, Weatherwax T, et al. Blood Occludin level as a potential biomarker for early blood brain barrier damage following ischemic stroke. Scientific Reports. 2017;**7**:40331

[45] Li W, Qi Z, Kang H, et al. Serum occludin as a biomarker to predict the severity of acute ischemic stroke, hemorrhagic transformation, and patient prognosis. Aging and Disease. 2020;**11**:1395-1406

[46] Beroun A, Mitra S, Michaluk P, et al. MMPs in learning and memory and neuropsychiatric disorders. Cellular and Molecular Life Sciences : CMLS. 2019;**76**:3207-3228

[47] Van Doren SR. Matrix metalloproteinase interactions with collagen and elastin. Matrix Biology : Journal of the International Society for Matrix Biology. 2015;**44-46**:224-231

[48] Yuan J, Zhang Y, Zhang Y, et al. Effects of metal nanoparticles on tight junction-associated proteins via HIF-1α/miR-29b/MMPs pathway in human epidermal keratinocytes. Particle and Fibre Toxicology. 2021;**18**:13

[49] Chen F, Hori T, Ohashi N, et al. Occludin is regulated by epidermal growth factor receptor activation in brain endothelial cells and brains of mice with acute liver failure. Hepatology [Baltimore, Md.]. 2011;**53**:1294-1305

[50] Nelson PT, Dickson DW, Trojanowski JQ, et al. Limbic-predominant age-related TDP-43 encephalopathy [LATE]: Consensus working group report. Brain : A Journal of Neurology. 2019;**142**:1503-1527

[51] Behzadian MA, Wang XL, Windsor LJ, et al. TGF-beta increases retinal endothelial cell permeability by increasing MMP-9: Possible role of glial cells in endothelial barrier function. Investigative Ophthalmology & Visual Science. 2001;**42**:853-859

[52] Bauer AT, Bürgers HF, Rabie T, et al. Matrix metalloproteinase-9 mediates hypoxia-induced vascular leakage in the brain via tight junction rearrangement. Journal of Cerebral Blood Flow and Metabolism: Official Journal of the International Society of Cerebral Blood Flow and Metabolism. 2010;**30**:837-848

[53] Chen W, Hartman R, Ayer R, et al. Matrix metalloproteinases inhibition provides neuroprotection against hypoxia-ischemia in the developing brain. Journal of Neurochemistry. 2009;**111**:726-736

[54] Lischper M, Beuck S, Thanabalasundaram G, et al. Metalloproteinase mediated occludin cleavage in the cerebral microcapillary endothelium under pathological

conditions. Brain Research. 2010;**1326**:114-127

[55] Tada Y, Yagi K, Kitazato KT, et al. Reduction of endothelial tight junction proteins is related to cerebral aneurysm formation in rats. Journal of Hypertension. 2010;**28**:1883-1891

[56] Giebel SJ, Menicucci G, McGuire PG, et al. Matrix metalloproteinases in early diabetic retinopathy and their role in alteration of the blood-retinal barrier. Laboratory Investigation; A Journal of Technical Methods and Pathology. 2005;**85**:597-607

[57] Hawkins BT, Lundeen TF, Norwood KM, et al. Increased blood-brain barrier permeability and altered tight junctions in experimental diabetes in the rat: Contribution of hyperglycaemia and matrix metalloproteinases. Diabetologia. 2007;**50**:202-211

[58] Caron A, Desrosiers RR, Langlois S, et al. Ischemia-reperfusion injury stimulates gelatinase expression and activity in kidney glomeruli. Canadian Journal of Physiology and Pharmacology. 2005;**83**:287-300

[59] Ishihara H, Kubota H, Lindberg RL, et al. Endothelial cell barrier impairment induced by glioblastomas and transforming growth factor beta2 involves matrix metalloproteinases and tight junction proteins. Journal of Neuropathology and Experimental Neurology. 2008;**67**:435-448

[60] Lohmann C, Krischke M, Wegener J, et al. Tyrosine phosphatase inhibition induces loss of blood-brain barrier integrity by matrix metalloproteinase-dependent and -independent pathways. Brain Research. 2004;**995**:184-196

[61] Wan H, Winton HL, Soeller C, et al. Quantitative structural and biochemical analyses of tight junction dynamics following exposure of epithelial cells to house dust mite allergen Der p 1. Clinical and Experimental Allergy: Journal of the British Society for Allergy and Clinical Immunology. 2000;**30**:685-698

[62] Bojarski C, Weiske J, Schöneberg T, et al. The specific fates of tight junction proteins in apoptotic epithelial cells. Journal of Cell Science. 2004;**117**:2097-2107

[63] Bilbrough T, Piemontese E, Seitz O. Dissecting the role of protein phosphorylation: A chemical biology toolbox. Chemical Society Reviews. 2022;**51**:5691-5730

[64] Sakakibara A, Furuse M, Saitou M, et al. Possible involvement of phosphorylation of occludin in tight junction formation. The Journal of Cell Biology. 1997;**137**:1393-1401

[65] Farshori P, Kachar B. Redistribution and phosphorylation of occludin during opening and resealing of tight junctions in cultured epithelial cells. The Journal of Membrane Biology. 1999;**170**:147-156

[66] Tsukamoto T, Nigam SK. Role of tyrosine phosphorylation in the reassembly of occludin and other tight junction proteins. The American Journal of Physiology. 1999;**276**:F737-F750

[67] Dörfel MJ, Westphal JK, Bellmann C, et al. CK2-dependent phosphorylation of occludin regulates the interaction with ZO-proteins and tight junction integrity. Cell Communication and Signaling : CCS. 2013;**11**:40

[68] Goncalves A, Dreffs A, Lin CM, et al. Vascular expression of permeability-resistant occludin mutant preserves visual function in diabetes. Diabetes. 2021;**70**:1549-1560

[69] András IE, Deli MA, Veszelka S, et al. The NMDA and AMPA/KA receptors are involved in glutamate-induced alterations of occludin expression and phosphorylation in brain endothelial cells. Journal of Cerebral Blood Flow and Metabolism : Official Journal of the International Society of Cerebral Blood Flow and Metabolism. 2007;**27**:1431-1443

[70] Yamamoto M, Ramirez SH, Sato S, et al. Phosphorylation of claudin-5 and occludin by rho kinase in brain endothelial cells. The American Journal of Pathology. 2008;**172**:521-533

[71] Seth A, Sheth P, Elias BC, et al. Protein phosphatases 2A and 1 interact with occludin and negatively regulate the assembly of tight junctions in the CACO-2 cell monolayer. The Journal of Biological Chemistry. 2007;**282**:11487-11498

[72] Suzuki T, Elias BC, Seth A, et al. PKC eta regulates occludin phosphorylation and epithelial tight junction integrity. Proceedings of the National Academy of Sciences of the United States of America. 2009;**106**:61-66

[73] Popovic D, Vucic D, Dikic I. Ubiquitination in disease pathogenesis and treatment. Nature Medicine. 2014;**20**:1242-1253

[74] Shaid S, Brandts CH, Serve H, et al. Ubiquitination and selective autophagy. Cell Death and Differentiation. 2013;**20**:21-30

[75] Traweger A, Fang D, Liu YC, et al. The tight junction-specific protein occludin is a functional target of the E3 ubiquitin-protein ligase itch. The Journal of Biological Chemistry. 2002;**277**:10201-10208

[76] Lui WY, Lee WM. cAMP perturbs inter-Sertoli tight junction permeability barrier in vitro via its effect on proteasome-sensitive ubiquitination of occludin. Journal of Cellular Physiology. 2005;**203**:564-572

[77] Raikwar NS, Vandewalle A, Thomas CP. Nedd4-2 interacts with occludin to inhibit tight junction formation and enhance paracellular conductance in collecting duct epithelia. American Journal of Physiology. Renal Physiology. 2010;**299**:F436-F444

[78] Murakami T, Felinski EA, Antonetti DA. Occludin phosphorylation and ubiquitination regulate tight junction trafficking and vascular endothelial growth factor-induced permeability. The Journal of Biological Chemistry. 2009;**284**:21036-21046

[79] Tang J, Kang Y, Zhou Y, et al. ALS-causing SOD1 mutants regulate occludin phosphorylation/ubiquitination and endocytic trafficking via the ITCH/Eps15/Rab5 axis. Neurobiology of Disease. 2021;**153**:105315

[80] Zhang GS, Tian Y, Huang JY, et al. The γ-secretase blocker DAPT reduces the permeability of the blood-brain barrier by decreasing the ubiquitination and degradation of occludin during permanent brain ischemia. CNS Neuroscience & Therapeutics. 2013;**19**:53-60

[81] Rom S, Heldt NA, Gajghate S, Seliga A, Reichenbach NL, Persidsky Y. Hyperglycemia and advanced glycation end products disrupt BBB and promote occludin and claudin-5 protein secretion on extracellular microvesicles. Scientific Reports. 2020;**10**(1):7274

[82] Nikolian VC, Dekker SE, Bambakidis T, Higgins GA, Dennahy IS, Georgoff PE, et al. Improvement of blood-brain barrier integrity in traumatic brain injury and hemorrhagic shock

following treatment with valproic acid and fresh frozen plasma. Critical Care Medicine. 2018;**46**(1):e59-e66

[83] Kim KA, Kim D, Kim JH, Shin YJ, Kim ES, Akram M, et al. Autophagy-mediated occludin degradation contributes to blood-brain barrier disruption during ischemia in bEnd.3 brain endothelial cells and rat ischemic stroke models. Fluids Barriers CNS. 2020;**171**:21

[84] Zhang Y, Li X, Qiao S, Yang D, Li Z, Xu J, et al. Occludin degradation makes brain microvascular endothelial cells more vulnerable to reperfusion injury *in vitro*. Journal of Neurochemistry. 2021;**156**(3):352-366

[85] Ogata S, Ito S, Masuda T, Ohtsuki S. Changes of blood-brain barrier and brain parenchymal protein expression levels of mice under different insulin-resistance conditions induced by high-fat diet. Pharmaceutical Research. 2019;**36**(10):141

[86] Higashi Y, Sukhanov S, Shai SY, Danchuk S, Snarski P, Li Z, et al. Endothelial deficiency of insulin-like growth factor-1 receptor reduces endothelial barrier function and promotes atherosclerosis in Apoe-deficient mice. American Journal of Physiology. Heart and Circulatory Physiology. 2020;**319**(4):H730-H743

[87] Good RB, Gilbane AJ, Trinder SL, Denton CP, Coghlan G, Abraham DJ, et al. Endothelial to mesenchymal transition contributes to endothelial dysfunction in pulmonary arterial hypertension. The American Journal of Pathology. 2015;**185**(7):1850-1858

[88] Lee JH, Chinnathambi A, Alharbi SA, Shair OHM, Sethi G, Ahn KS. Farnesol abrogates epithelial to mesenchymal transition process through regulating Akt/mTOR pathway. Pharmacological Research. 2019;**150**:104504

[89] Liu H, Gu C, Liu M, Liu G, Wang D, Liu X, et al. Ventilator-induced lung injury is alleviated by inhibiting NLRP3 inflammasome activation. Molecular Immunology. 2019;**111**:1-10

[90] Lee SY, Shin JA, Kwon HM, Weiner ID, Han KH. Renal ischemia-reperfusion injury causes intercalated cell-specific disruption of occludin in the collecting duct. Histochemistry and Cell Biology. 2011;**136**(6):637-647

[91] Yin Q, Xia Y, Wang G. Sinomenine alleviates high glucose-induced renal glomerular endothelial hyperpermeability by inhibiting the activation of RhoA/ROCK signaling pathway. Biochemical and Biophysical Research Communications. 2016;**477**(4):881-886

[92] Gonzalez A, Krieg R, Massey HD, Carl D, Ghosh S, Gehr TWB, et al. Sodium butyrate ameliorates insulin resistance and renal failure in CKD rats by modulating intestinal permeability and mucin expression. Nephrology, Dialysis, Transplantation. 2019;**34**(5):783-794

[93] Zhang T, Ouyang H, Mei X, Lu B, Yu Z, Chen K, et al. Erianin alleviates diabetic retinopathy by reducing retinal inflammation initiated by microglial cells via inhibiting hyperglycemia-mediated ERK1/2-NF-κB signaling pathway. The FASEB Journal. 2019;**33**(11):11776-11790

[94] Rathnasamy G, Sivakumar V, Foulds WS, Ling EA, Kaur C. Vascular changes in the developing rat retina in response to hypoxia. Experimental Eye Research. 2015;**130**:73-86

[95] Wu Y, Meng R, Rajah GB, Ding Y, Xu Y, Ji X. Blood-brain barrier disruption

may contribute to white matter lesions in the setting of internal jugular venous stenosis. Current Neurovascular Research. 2019;**16**(4):328-334

[96] Nitta K, Nishinaka A, Hida Y, Nakamura S, Shimazawa M, Hara H. Oral and ocular administration of crocetin prevents retinal edema in a murine retinal vein occlusion model. Molecular Vision. 2019;**25**:859-868

[97] Chai J, Long B, Liu X, Li Y, Han N, Zhao P, et al. Effects of sevoflurane on tight junction protein expression and PKC-α translocation after pulmonary ischemia-reperfusion injury. Experimental & Molecular Medicine. 2015;**47**(6):e167

Section 3

Endothelial Dysfunction: A Clinical Correlate

Chapter 5

Endothelial Dysfunction in Appendicitis

Erjan Fikri, Ahmad Razi Maulana Alnaz and Fini Meirisa Alnaz

Abstract

In an inflammation, including appendicitis, vascular adequacy is required to supply anti-inflammatory substances and nutrition due to inflamed tissue remodeling. Normal tissue has balanced tissue regeneration and tissue destruction from apoptosis. While in inflammation, inflammatory substances tend to cause tissue destruction and lead to necrosis. This requires the tissue to increase cell regeneration to maintain tissue homeostasis in the appendix, induced mainly by oxygenation, nutrition, growth factors, and mainly anti-inflammatory substances that are obtained with vascular adequacy. This process needs active vascularization that can be achieved with neovascularization to ensure good vascularization to the tissue lacking from vascular damage. The ability of neovascularization is mainly related to growth factors acting in the endothelium and inducing neovascularization process. This mechanism is impaired in the process of inflammation by inflammatory substances causing endothelial dysfunction. As stated that vascular adequacy is related to growth factors such as vascular endothelial growth factors (VEGF) that may differ from one person to another, external and internal factors plays role in affecting individualized difference in adapting to inflammatory process, the expression of the VEGF may be a novel distinction to cut-off requirements of inflammation process in appendicitis would be self-limiting or continue to cause tissue necrosis and perforating appendicitis that urges surgical treatment to encounter the unstoppable inflammatory process in the appendix.

Keywords: appendicitis, endothelial dysfunction, inflammation, neovascularization, VEGF

1. Introduction

Appendicitis is an inflammation of the vermiform appendix, which presents as one of the causes of acute abdomen leading to emergency surgical indication. The acute appendicitis presented as the most common indication of nontraumatic emergency surgeries around the world. Annually, more than 100 cases of appendicitis per 100,000 persons are recorded around the world. About 16.33% of men and 16.34% of women mostly in the second and third decades of life were at risk of experiencing acute appendicitis [1, 2].

IntechOpen

More than 108,000 surgical procedures were conducted to treat appendicitis in a year. Acute appendicitis may be treated with surgical treatment and conservative treatment. Treatment choices were considered in acute appendicitis by classification of clinical uncomplicated or complicated appendicitis occurred [3].

Distinguishing indications of surgery or appendectomy as treatment of appendicitis might be challenging. It was more subtle in pediatric patients, as more consideration and careful examination needed to be conducted prior to the surgical procedure. Statistics had recorded more events of negative appendectomy, the fact that vermiform appendix presented to be normal or not inflamed after the process of appendectomy. The incidence was commonly only about 15% in adults but raised up to 56.7% or even more in pediatric patients presenting with related symptoms to appendicitis. These procedures were stated as a burden in medical decision-making as non-indicative surgeries may harm patients or even cause expenditures for non-beneficial procedures [4].

The main aim of diagnostic and decision-making in appendicitis was to accurately distinguish any chance of currently symptomatic appendicitis appearing normal as presented during operation. This means that appendicitis may be reversible and basic inflammation of the appendicitis was not causing permanent damage to the appendix vermiform itself. Currently, there was still no such strong evidence to prove whether an appendicitis process that occurred would end as permanent tissue damage and causes complications that are mandatory for surgical treatment of the appendix vermiform or would heal without risk of complications [5].

We analyzed the possibilities of differentiation of the two conditions in appendicitis. The main key to understand and accurately differentiate risk in appendicitis would be clearly explained in a basic inflammatory mechanism on how appendicitis would occur. The promising approach was glancing at the pathways and mechanism of inflammation would occur specifically, as related with factors lying alongside the pathophysiological process of inflammation and cure of the inflammation itself, by sufficient oxygenation and adequate metabolism of remodeling or tissue repair.

2. The appendix vermiformis

The appendix vermiform is an anatomical structure located at the end of cecum, commonly in posteromedial projection, located about 1.7 cm below the ileocecal valve, at the end of the taenias of the colon converging on the cecum. Its size is about 91.2 mm long in men and 80.3 mm in women, respectively. The appendix is a true diverticulum, as its layer is made up of mucosa, submucosa, longitudinal and circular muscle, and serosa. Anatomically, the position of the appendix just located anterior to the iliopsoas muscle and the lumbar plexus, and posterior to the layers of abdominal wall muscles. The main blood supply to the appendix comes from the appendicular artery, one branch of ileocolic artery, which extends along the mesoappendix to the distal tip of the appendix. Mesoappendix is a mesenterium consists of connective tissue anchoring the appendix into the mesentery of the intestines which size varies to the size of the appendix itself. Somehow, angle and projection of the appendix may differ from one to another: retrocecal, subcecal, preileal, postileal, and pelvic (**Figure 1**) [6, 7].

Nutrition of the vermiform appendix was obtained by special vessels vasculating the appendix running along the mesoappendix. Main nutrition and oxygenation living the appendix are supplied by the appendicular artery, derived and branched from the ileocolic artery alongside the ileum, cecum, and ascending colon. The

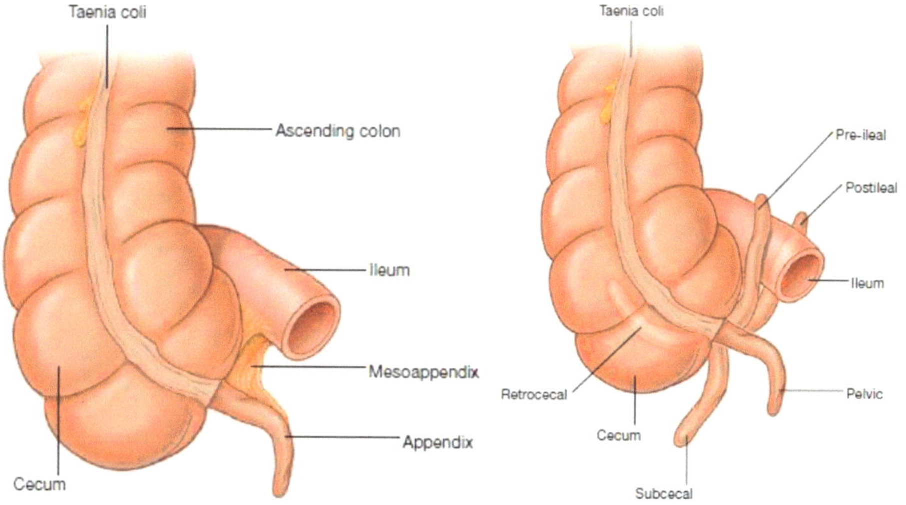

Figure 1.
The anatomy of vermiform appendix and the cecum (left) and its anatomical variations (right) [6].

appendicular artery was 1 single branch from the ileocolic artery vascularize the whole appendix which then performed networks of smaller arteries perforating into the layers of appendix. The vascularization of the appendix originates from mesenteric blood circulation which is also responsible for other parts of the intestinal circulation. The appendicular artery is one of the most distal parts of the branches from the superior mesenteric circulation. Although it is part of the huge mesenteric circulation, as appendiceal circulation took a little part and branch among the circulation, the regulation of blood flow is less and lower than in other parts of the mesenteric circulation such as in the ileum or ascending colon. However, regulation of the blood flow is commonly maintained by local factors with vasodilator effects induced and attributed by hypoxia or cytokines of inflammation to cause an increase in blood flow to the appendix. Certain osmotic mechanisms, autonomic and neurohumoral, also the intestinal wall activity of peristalsis affect the blood flow in the mesenteric circulation primarily the special circulation to the appendix [6, 8].

Metabolic end products from the tissue in the vermiform appendix were drained away by the venous drainage which anatomically will join the venous blood flow in the ileocolic vein and the superior mesenteric vein. Another non-venous drainage of the appendix occurs by the lymphatic drainage of the cecum and the appendix which passes the lymph nodes in the mesoappendix and ileocolic lymph nodes surrounding the ileocolic artery into a group of superior mesenteric lymph nodes (**Figure 2**) [9].

The vermiform appendix is known as a vestigial organ embryologically and by the evolution of mammals. The main functions of vermiform appendicitis itself remain unknown. Theories stated that in humans the vermiform appendix no longer functions but other theories counters. As histologically it is rich in lymphoid tissue and its vascularization and lymphatics, its function is mostly discussed related to the immunological functions, especially to the gastrointestinal system. As its luminal and non-continuous structure, the vermiform appendix was also hypothesized to be a reservoir for gut microbiota. This function and structure were suspected to have strong correlations to inflammatory mediators and microbiological mechanisms of the bacteria.

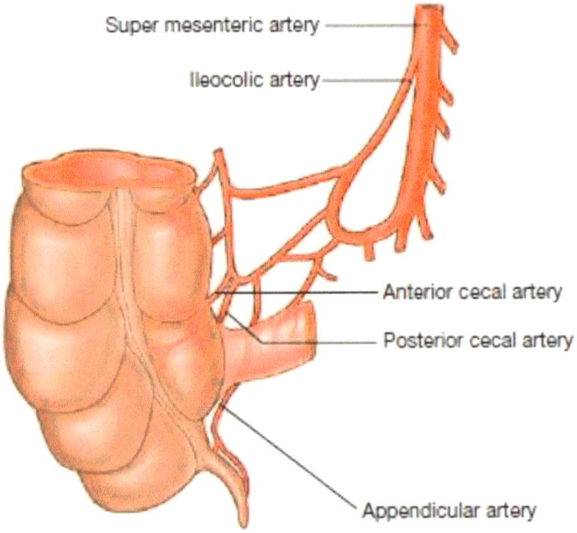

Figure 2.
Arterial supply of the vermiform appendix [6].

This puts the vermiform appendix as an organ with a lot of risks of inflammations and infections its homeostasis was disrupted [10].

3. Appendicitis

Appendicitis is defined as inflammation of the vermiform appendix and represents the most common cause of acute abdomen and emergency surgical indication in the world [1]. As common to all kinds of inflammation and precisely to the gut, appendicitis was commonly related to biochemical, histological, and physiological changes to the vermiform appendix itself. Inflammatory mediators regardless of factors precipitating lead to common manifest of inflammatory signs of a fluid shift, size changes (enlargement), increased blood flow and perfusion, inflammatory cell infiltrations, and also tissue remodeling, especially to the lymphoid tissues of the appendix. The inflammatory process as occur in all tissue may be reversible and some tend to be permanent remodeling or end with tissue damage and causes complication of appendicitis [11].

Presentation of appendicitis occurs by luminal obstruction of the appendix lumen that may be precipitated by a variety of etiologies, whether due to mass, faecolith or appendicolith, mucosal inflammation, lymphoid tissue hyperplasia, parasite infestations, or other mechanism leading to disruption of the passage of fluid and any luminal contents in the appendix to be propelled away to the cecum, and causing maladaptive mechanism that started certain cascade of pathophysiological events of inflammation that would be manifested clinically [12].

Clinical manifestation of appendicitis may be challenging. Most common symptom that occurs and causes patients to seek medical care is abdominal pain, although other symptoms such as fever, constipation, diarrhea, anorexia, and nausea are also reported as the main symptom. Pain in appendicitis starts in periumbilical and epigastric region at the beginning of the onset, and later migrates to the lower right quadrant where classic McBurney sign of classic lower right quadrant pain occurs. However, the history of migratory pain from one to another abdominal region occurs only in 50–60% of patients with acute appendicitis. Symptoms of nausea and vomiting start as the effect of abdominal pain, and fever starts about 6 hours after the onset of pain where an inflammatory process in the appendix had been established. The history of symptoms may be different from one patient to another, related to the anatomical variation of the appendix. Anteriorly located appendix commonly causes more marked and localized pain in the right lower quadrant, and the variation of retro-cecal one commonly has a dull abdominal pain manifestation or may be interpreted as a lower lumbar region pain. Furthermore, as appendicitis occurs with inflammation not restricted only to the appendix itself but may affect surrounding organs, other symptoms such as urinary urgency, dysuria, or rectal symptoms may appear but some cases [13, 14].

Physical examinations of patients with appendicitis include basic vital sign findings followed by an appendicitis-specific examination. Patients with appendicitis mostly present as febrile with a temperature greater than 38°C, tachycardia, and tachypnea may be found. Most early clinical manifestation of appendicitis are mostly non-specific and mimics other gastrointestinal disturbances. Obvious manifestation would present when inflammation progresses when inflammation had involved the parietal peritoneum in the serosa of the appendix which causes localized right lower quadrant tenderness that further exacerbates by specific physical examination such as McBurney sign, Rovsig sign, or other signs of appendicitis. However, the pain would progress more to be exacerbated by movement or cough causing an increase in intraabdominal pressure. Routine laboratory test usually provides an increase in leukocytes, especially neutrophil as an acute reaction to the inflammatory process presents a shifting to the left in leukocyte differential count. C-reactive protein indicates that systemic inflammation with greater than 1.5 mg/l may be one of the likely diagnostic indicators of appendicitis [15].

Further complicated and severe appendicitis usually has leukocytosis counts more than 20,000/μl and commonly related to perforation dan peritonitis and high level of C-reactive protein or even Procalcitonin. However, perforation and complicated appendicitis were also reported in about 10% of appendicitis with normal to mild increase in leukocyte count and C-reactive protein. This could not exclude the possibility of perforation in normal laboratory values in appendicitis. This because low sensitivity of leukocyte count in the diagnosis of appendicitis with only 65–75% while only 57–87% for C-reactive protein. Therefore, many studies had been conducted on early specific diagnosis; such as procalcitonin, as it is a good biomarker in sepsis and appendicitis may lead to sepsis but is still limited in appendicitis with no sepsis [15].

3.1 Pathophysiology of appendicitis

Exact pathophysiology of appendicitis itself remains a struggle for physicians. The process of appendicitis itself is related and basically similar to other pathophysiology of inflammations. Commonly appendicitis began with a luminal obstruction. Several causes of obstruction may occur such as lymphoid hyperplasia, parasitic infections, fecalith, or intra and extra luminal mass. This causes an increase of intraluminal and intramural pressure which causes small vascular and lymphatic occlusion collapsed by the tension of the lumen and mural. Obstructed appendix tends to cause overgrowth of bacteria, mostly aerobic bacteria dominate in acute appendicitis [16].

The obstruction may also cause mucous plaques and accumulated causing distension. Distension of the appendix may progress vary from one patient to another up to 50–65 mmHg. When the luminal pressure increases, vascularization in the mural may be disrupted. Increase in the pressure may beyond the lymphatic and venous pressure and prevents fluid drain from the two vessels due to a weak wall of vein and lymphatics [17]. First collapsed vessel would be the lymphatic drainage preventing fluid back into circulation to remain in the appendix tissue. Soon as pressure increases in the lumen, the pressure disrupted the lumen of the vein and causes collapse of both lymph and blood flow from the tissue of the appendix. This process causes the edema process which occurred by disrupted fluid drainage [14, 18].

This state of appendicitis consisted of inflammation and edema alone possibly start the clinical symptoms of appendicitis, but this stage is considered as a mild process in which conservative treatment for appendicitis may be available. Surgical treatment may be offered, and still may be beneficial but as it is an invasive procedure and has a number of complications, the surgical procedure which is still not yet urgent to be performed may not be a favorable choice of treatment. Antibiotics and good fiber intake may be one of the choice and helps relieve symptoms and reduce the inflammation of appendicitis [5, 19].

But the mild state of appendicitis also has a risk to develop further. Fluid accumulation and edema also cause more tension to the vascular wall causing further obstruction and disruptions of vessel flows. Soon as the pressure increases more the arterial walls were collapsed due to pressure to its wall. The blood flow containing oxygens and nutrients was decreased due to arterial obstructions. This stated the condition of hypoxia in the distal of the arterial obstruction in the appendix [20].

Hypoxia state of the mucosa and the wall of the appendix begins further tissue damage in the appendix. Tissue damages were due to hypoxic stress of the cells in the appendix which then undergo a cell apoptosis process of even necrosis of the tissue. Tissue damage causes less strength of the appendix wall from distensions of the edema and fluid accumulation that is then related to complications by ulcerations, perforations, and necrotic appendix. This process occurs only if the vascularization were disrupted. Hypoxic environment also tends to be favorable for growth of intestinal flora mostly the Gram-negative bacterias such as *Escherichia coli, Enterococcus, Bacteroides,* and *Pseudomonas*. Bacterial growth also elicits more inflammatory and immunologic processes in the appendix itself. *E. coli* itself as the main flora normal in the large intestine may cause activity changes and be pathogenic as shifted and trapped in the appendix with different microenvironments and releases toxins exacerbates inflammation [13, 20].

The tissue damage and necrosis in appendicitis risk a thin and fragile wall of the appendix. This at one point with more pressure would lead to a tear of the mucosal or even the muscular and serous layer of the wall causing perforation of the appendix. Once a perforation occur, acute appendicitis occurred with complication. As bacterial overgrowth inside the lumen of the appendix came in contact with the sterile peritoneum cavity begins further immune and inflammatory responses cause peritonitis. As peritonitis occurred in complicated appendicitis, operative treatment with laparotomy may be inevitable. Further inflammatory process of the peritoneal wall also risks the spread of bacteria into the bloodstream and may complicate more into sepsis with all its high risk of mortality [21, 22].

Bacterial growth causes inflammation, especially in the mucosa of the appendix. The incompetence of the appendiceal wall risk the development of spreading infections and inflammatory mediators causing inflammation of the serous layer of the appendix. A close anatomical layer of the serous into the parietal peritoneum and other adjacent organs. The inflammation of the peritoneum led to appendicitis complicated with peritonitis. Stimulation of pain fibers of the afferent visceral pain nerves in the layer of the peritoneum to the level of medulla spinalis. Pain sensation is interpreted as epigastric and periumbilical pain, which quality could not be specifically localized, but the right lower quadrant has the most accumulation of inflammatory mediators that would inflame more and be more painful [12, 20].

Untreated and uncompensated process of inflammation leads the more serious complications of appendicitis. The longer the hypoxia occurs to the tissue, the more risk of tissue damage. Risk of infarction multiplied by time followed by progression into perforated or even gangrenous appendicitis. More severe symptoms as mentioned previously would progress and limits daily activity. More pain and nausea and vomiting would occur. Systemic involvement in sepsis may be part of the risk of prolonged appendicitis. The process and pathophysiology off appendicitis may be illustrated in **Figure 3** [16, 22].

Basically, no major changes occur in mesenteric circulation in appendicitis. However, as a reaction to inflammation, local vascularization specifically targeting the inflamed tissue increased and was hypothesized to activate the neovascularization in the collateral circulations nearby mucosa and muscular layer of the appendix. The tiny new collateral vasculature along the local inflammation we aimed to increase perfusion into the center of inflammation, which is highly fragile and requires

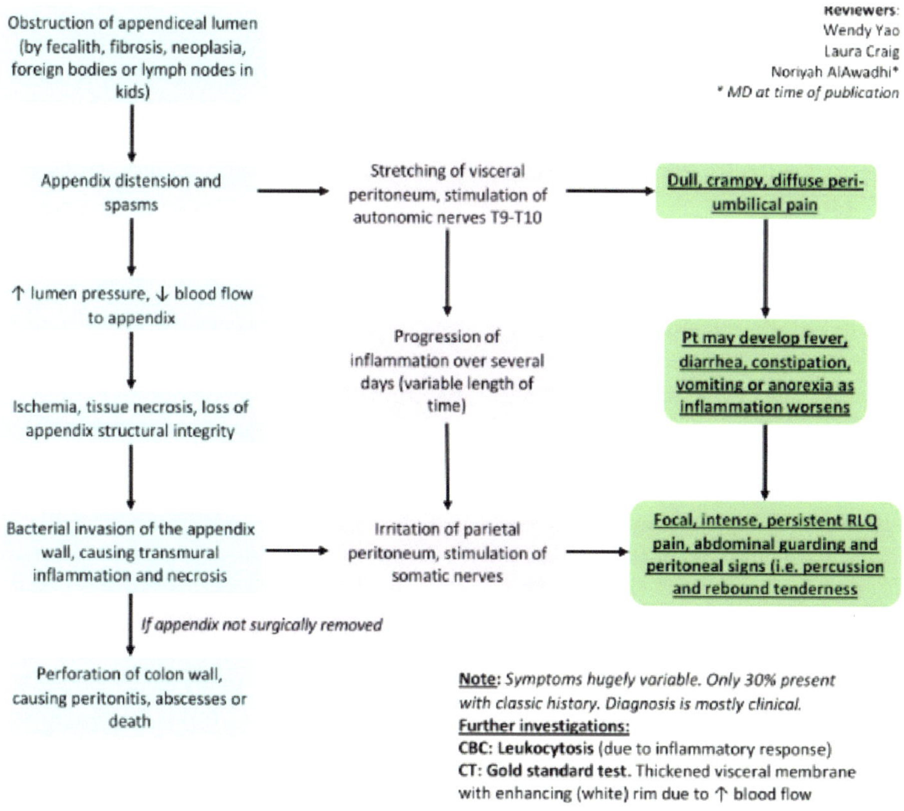

Figure 3.
The pathophysiology of appendicitis [23].

strong endothelial stability which may be supported by certain endothelial factors to maintain perfusion against high intraluminal pressure from the appendix itself and preventing collapsed or burst of the vascularization [23, 24].

Severity and complications of appendicitis are known to be related with necrosis or ischemic tissue in the appendix vermiform. Basic consideration on factors affecting the vascularization patency to tissue damage in appendicitis. Arteries with dysfunctioned endothelium occasionally damaged and unable to adapt and perform potent perfusion to tissues in systemic changes caused by the inflammatory mediators. While arteries with good endothelium tend to be able to keep strong perfusion to maintain oxygenation preventing cell death. This differentiates variations of symptoms in patients with appendicitis who develops complication and whom did not [25].

This means mucosal vascularization of the appendix was considered as a barrier preventing further damage to the mucosa from increased intraluminal pressure in appendicitis. So as the mucosal and muscular layer of the appendix receives adequate vascularization, tissue elasticity and cell regeneration would take place so that the tissue would able to adapt against stretch elicited by the increase of the intraluminal pressure. Furthermore, enough perfusion to the appendiceal muscular layer will be able to initiate appendiceal contractility to drain out fluid or any fecalith obstructing and causing trapped intraluminal contain. This tissue competence may be a key role in preventing the perforation of other complications of appendicitis [26].

3.2 Recovery process in appendicitis

The appendix as a rich in lymphoid tissue part of the intestine has a high reserve of natural killer cells (NK)111 CD31 T cells (NK T lymphocytes). This cell produces cytokines and chemokines early since activated by the local inflammatory process. Cells such as B2201CD31 T cells in the lymphoid of the appendix express CD45R indicates for T cell activations more than any part of the intestine. Certain factors related to a great number of lymphocytes in the appendix came as the presence of CCL21, a chemokine embedded to the lymphatic endothelial cells and luminal surface of endothelial venules around the parafollicular areas in MALT. CCL21 binds to CCR7 to promote recruitment of B and T lymphocytes to the appendiceal lymphoid tissue and migration of dendritic cells (DC) back to appendiceal lymph nodes [15].

Apart from the abundant lymphocytes in the appendix, the molecular expression on the surface of the lymphocytes in the appendix differs from lymphocytes in the intestinal lymphocytes. In the lamina propria, the T cells in the lamina propria of the appendix express more integrin subunit b7 than B cells and also than the lymphocytes in the other parts of the intestine. Integrin a4b7 is expressed on T cells located between lamina propria and epithelium, and on macrophages and dendritic cells located in the mucosa of the appendix [22]. The molecule binds to mucosal addressin cell adhesion molecule 1 (MAdCAM-1), which mediation process of "tethering and rolling" and "homing" attracts lymphocytes into it. The localized expression of these molecules of a4b7 is considered a trafficking signal. Conversely, the aEb7 is responsible for the retention of these lymphocytes, via binding with its ligand E-cadherin. The dendritic cells express aEb7 stimulate the differentiation of forkhead box protein 3 (FoxP3)1 Treg cells soon after the interactions with antigens. Therefore, the suppression of regulatory expression would prevent lymphocyte differentiation and lead to a proinflammatory state [14].

CD51 cells or B1 lymphocytes are expressed more in a healthy appendix than the rest of the gut. When the appendix inflamed, the expression increased even more. These CD51 B cells produce IgM antibodies specific to certain pathogens. The synthesis of the IgM could take place directly in case of the absence of antigen presentation by other T cells, similar to innate-like immune response expressed by IELs. Despite the ability to synthesize IgM similar to immune response, the IgM antigen has low affinities, it still has major importance in reaction to microorganisms. Increase in the expression would be explained by an alteration of the intestinal microflora that occurs along the pathogenesis of appendicitis. Moreover, the CD51 cells also produce anti-self antibodies and an anti-inflammatory molecule such as IL-10 which means the increase of the expression was process to prevent inflammation currently occurring [27].

Pathologically, the complications of appendicitis were affected by the mucosal resistance to stress and adequate vascularity (microvessel density) in the appendix mucosa. This prevents further tissue damage. The mucosal resistance is determined by its adequacy to regenerate in case of stress or damage, producing new and strong mucosal layer which is influenced by folic acid (FA) metabolism. Adequate vascularity is then determined by ability of angiogenesis which plays as on of the most important factors in wound healing process. The angiogenesis itself is induced by growth factors namely vascular endothelial growth factor (VEGF), which role is fundamental by mediating and inducing the neovascularization, reepithelialization, and regulation of extracellular matrix. However the VEGF expression itself is endothelial cells in the blood vessels [28].

The angiogenesis occurs and induced in appendicitis, forming novel microvasculatures around the inflamed appendix to sustain adequate perfusion. The formation of new vascularization is required undergo the increased tissue's requirement of oxygen and nutrients of parenchymal remodeling, as well as to repair damaged blood vessels induced by pressure of inflammatory cytokines. Angiogenesis itself depends on VEGF, which is produced by damaged endothelial cells that stimulates mitosis in the endothelial lining of blood vessels creating new blood vessels other than currently damages vessel. This mechanism relates the VGEF to be believed associated with complicated appendicitis. Further evidence presented that different expression of VEGF may be found on histopathological examination of microvessel density in appendicitis specimens [28, 29].

Differentiating between risk of having complication may be a cut off on physician to take a concise decision on therapy of the patient. Patient which endothel may be strong enough responding the inflammatory process may not need to undergo operative treatment as tissue repair and remodeling were likely. However in chronic inflammation and weak endothelium possess a risk of further harm and requires surgical procedure [4, 12, 25].

Factors determining endothelial stabilities are regarding on tissue strength itself. Subgroup of individuals who tend to have a strong connective tissue subtypes of collagens has a chance to have a stronger endothelial stability. Factors effecting the endothelial growth and proliferations subsequently backs-up cells of the endothel to proliferate in preventing the endothelial damage. Also neovascularization may occur and possibly perfuse other sites of inflamed tissue to receive strong and supports of the vascularization. This prevents further complications to occur and more invasive treatment procedure may not be required or indicated as if antibiotics are capable [4, 19, 30]. The growth factor such as the vascular endothelial growth factor (VEGF) has a main role determining the strength of the endothelium against inflammation, especially in cases of appendicitis itself in the vascularization of the appendix [31].

4. Vascular endothelial growth factor (VEGF)

Vascular endothelial growth factor (VEGF, now referred to as VEGF-A) is a member of a family of proteins including VEGF-B, VEGF-C, VEGF-D, VEGF-E (virally encoded), and PlGF. VEGF-C and VEGF-D are primarily implicated in regulation of lymph angiogenesis. Given the dominant role that VEGF-A plays in regulating angiogenesis and disease, it will be referred to as VEGF. VEGF undergoes multiple splicing alternative creating several exon leading to multiple isoforms. Common isoforms include VEGF 165, VEGF 206, VEGF121, and VEGF189. VEGF165 (VEGF164 in mice) is the most frequently expressed isoform in majority of tissues. The VEGF165 is also the most physiologic isoform, with characteristics connected to the highly diffusible VEGF121 and the extracellular matrix (ECM)-bound VEGF189 [32, 33].

Less other isoforms of VEGF, such as VEGF145 and VEGF183 currently been described in several studies. Main features differentiates one isoforms than another were differential ability to bind heparin. The lowest affinity to heparin belongs to VEGF121, while strong affinity known for VEGF189 and VEGF206 which consist of two heparin-binding domains (encoded by exons 6 and 7), that may also bind to protein in the cell surfaces or the ECM. The most common VEGF165 has an intermediate binding ability with a single heparin-binding domain, encoded by exon 7, and has ability for ECM bound. In inflammatory process such as appendicitis, several proinflammatory molecules with protease ability such as the MMP3 and plasmin may alter the binding site of VEGF primarily at the COOH terminus and turns VEGF from ECM-bound peptides into non-heparin-binding, diffusible, molecular species which leads to less ability inducing angiogenesis [32].

Several inhibitory isoforms of VEGF have also been recently described, including VEGF165b and VEGFAx, but there is some controversy regarding the mechanisms of inhibition, and VEGF-Ax has now been shown to actually have pro-angiogenic and pro-permeability features. VEGF expression is majorly regulated by the hypoxia state by a transcription factor named hypoxia-inducible factor (HIF). The HIF and other genes related and activated by hypoxia plays role in diverse contexts activating several transcription of other growth factors including platelet-derived growth factor (PDGF), epidermal growth factor (EGF), and some oncogenic gene mutations (RAS, VHL, WNT-KRAS signaling pathway genes) which may control the VEGF expression in other side alters the VEGF-driven signaling [31].

The most understood VEGF signaling now is through VEGFR1/R2 regulation which controls the activities of several kinases and activation of its cascades to promote cell proliferation, survival, migration, and even influencing vascular permeability on angiogenesis. The endothelial cell, which consist of both tip and stalk cells are at the main site of vascular proliferation. VEGF gradients induce tip cells and promote the formation of filopodia. The molecular regulation of these events is via activation of notch signaling and by increased expression of notch ligands on endothelial cells, including but not limited to delta-like 4 (DLL4). The increased signaling of the notch in neighboring cells will reduces the expression of VEGFR2, which is causing a negative feedback loop to the signaling process. This main signaling pathway of the VEGF plays a critical role to maintain homeostasis, but as alteration of the pathway lead to hyperactivation by pathologic process leading to pathologic angiogenesis. Another pathway were described in 2014, named as a non-canonical pathway of VEGFR2 that was characterized in neurons. It is known to be expressed more in retinal neurons but are lacking in endothelial cells. Study reveals that a deletion gene responsible in

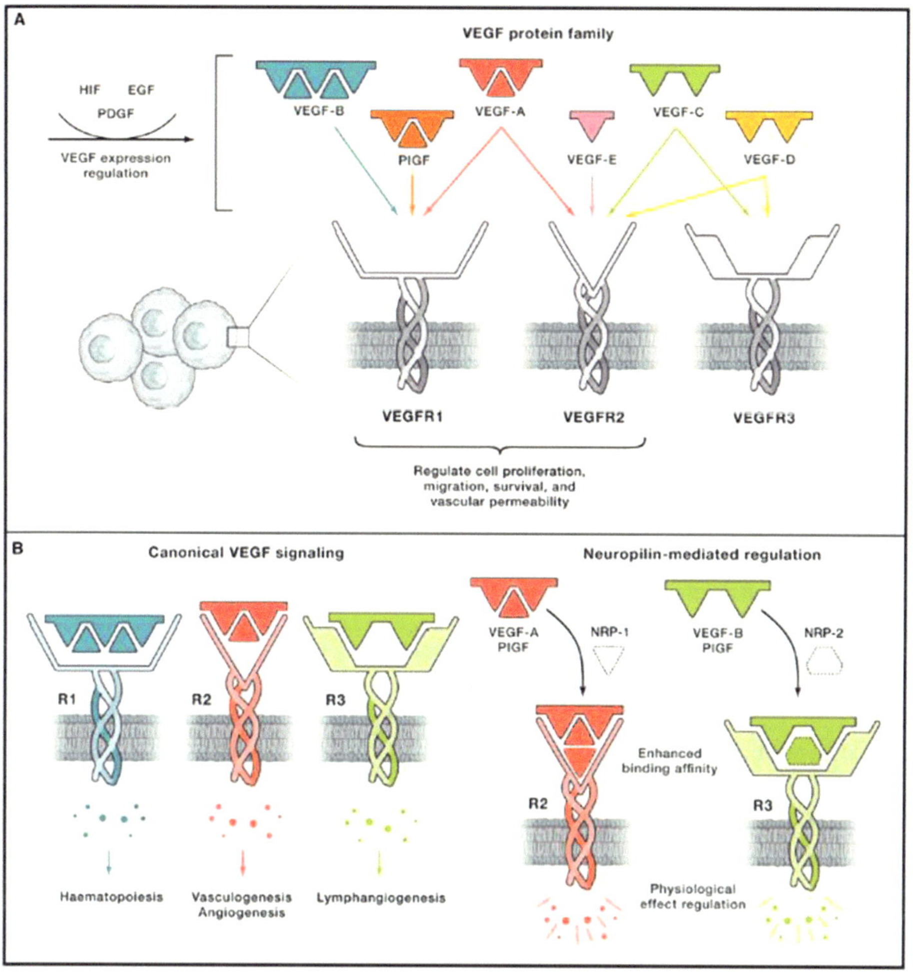

Figure 4.
VEGF activation and signaling pathways [33].

VEGFR2 pathway in neurons causes abnormal angiogenesis process by high VEGF expressions around the neuron tissue in response to deficiency of the VEGFR2. In other hand, the abnormal angiogenesis at the juxta-neural cells were common in response to maintain homeostasis in cases of ischemic retinopathy to ensure regenerative phase. This similar mechanism were a point of interest as number of VEGF expressed would be a critical factor to maintain tissue vascularization in several pathogenesis of tissue damage (**Figure 4**) [31, 33].

The findings that anti-VEGF antibodies decreased the growth of tumor cells implanted in immune-deficient mice opened up translational possibilities for targeting VEGF-VEGFR signaling. In addition, it was also demonstrated that inactivation of a single allele of the VEGF-A gene in mice resulted in defective vascular development and early embryonic lethality, highlighting the importance of VEGF during embryonic development. Inactivation of both copies of vegfr2 largely pheno-copied vegfa single-allele deletion. The ability to delete VEGF in target tissues with the advent of cre-lox systems created the possibility of assessing the role of VEGF in individual tissues/cells. Numerous studies employing this approach have documented the important role of VEGF in angiogenesis and homeostasis in a variety of pathophysiological circumstances [34].

4.1 Role of VEGF in appendicitis

Appendicitis is the most well-known gastrointestinal emergency and requires surgical approach in the pediatric population. The negative appendectomy rate is 8.4%, however largely higher among children aged <6 years at 56.7%. However, the diagnosis of appendicitis in children is often missed due even in a total examination. This article summarizes the current evidence on the influences of folic acid (FA) and vascular endothelial growth factor (VEGF) in appendicitis. The pathological processes of appendicitis could be approached by histopathological examination of microvessel thickness. Further analysis reveals that folic acid (FA) assumed a role in mucosal opposition and its capacity to recover, and VEGF (explicitly found in vein endothelial cells) was associated in tissue remodeling through a cycle of neovascularization, reepithelization, and guide of extracellular framework and has an important pro-angiogenic activity, having a mitogenic and an anti-apoptotic effect on endothelial cells, increasing the vascular permeability, promoting cell migration, etc. Due to these effects, it actively contributes in regulating the normal and pathological angiogenic processes [29].

Both folate acid and VEGF had a role as mentioned previously by certain cascades in the endothelial cells which may increase endothelial proliferation and induces branching of new collaterals during inflammation. This mechanism ensure enough and adequate blood flow locally around the appendix. The VEGF-induced proliferation among the endothelial cells adapts to race cell damages from stretch, cytokine induced cell death, and increase intraluminal pressures. This means collateral vascularization in the appendix were stabilized and able to receive more blood flow for tissue healing process. This puts VEGF has a special role in preventing tissue damage and the complication of appendicitis such as perforation or necrosis [35].

Folate acids had been widely concentrated in cardiovascular sickness and malignancy and an increased risk of infection among patients with insufficient degrees of folate acid. A low folate acid serum and raised homocysteine was shown to be found among patients with constant provocative infections and conditions such as systemic inflammatory illness and endothelial damage. A higher folate level would prevent endothelial damage as it would help maintain levels of homocysteine, vasodilators, and nitric oxide [28, 29, 36].

Similar patterns of reduction were also observed in basal VEGF levels among patients with appendicitis as reported by Fikri et al. However, the lower level in both FA and VEGF among patients with appendicitis were significant compared to control and a possible indicator in diagnosing complicated appendicitis. Another studies had reported increases in VEGF levels, namely in myocardial localized necrosis and was related to incendiary cytokines. The increasing levels of VEGF was directly associated with the number of hypoxia-inducible factors as it regulated the advancements of angiogenesis, vascular patency in atherogenic vessels. Fikri et al. further explained that VEGF levels in appendicitis has similar pattern as increase of VEGF during the stable phases after myocardial infarction and hence signifying that VEGF as a part of an ongoing inflammatory activity. The lower levels of VEGF often signifies a worsened condition and could be associated with a more complicated case of appendicitis [28, 36].

VEGF in conclusion, a histopathological examination of microvessel thickness is required to investigate the influences of FA and VEGF towards the pathological process of appendicitis among the pediatric population. Both FA and VEGF could be associated with disease progression where lower levels often indicated a more complicated case. A higher FA was associated with less provocative conditions with less inflammation and endothelial damage and a higher VEGF often suggested better prognosis as VEGF was used in angiogenesis etc. However, in both studies FA and VEGF were still limited of evidence as statistically significantly different towards controls in their use as a biomarker in the diagnosis complicated appendicitis were done in animals but human reaches are still conducted. However other factors regarding the endothelial functions in appendix are still limited to VEGF in current studies, other mechanism related to endothelin and the Fas-ligand were also in conduct for further evidence for the current update [26, 35].

5. Conclusions

Appendicitis is known as one of the most cause of emergency surgery. But beyond facts of its surgical emergency, basic pathophysiology of the appendicitis were not completely a surgical process. Manifestations and process of the inflammation of the appendicitis were also related to its vascularization and the stability of perfusion into the inflamed tissue. Factors contributing the quality of vascularization were consid ered to have a significant role in determining whether an appendicitis is a process of inflammation without or with complication, between non-surgical and surgical case. This fact may be guide further study physicians to differentiate indications of appendectomy and to be selectively careful and to reduce the number of negative appendectomies. Hance, current information and data were still provided by animal research model and laboratories studies, but rationally related to clinical manifests. However researches on the current topic with human sample of appendicitis is currently still conducted.

Conflict of interest

The author declared no conflict of interest in the process of writing this article.

Author details

Erjan Fikri[1*], Ahmad Razi Maulana Alnaz[2] and Fini Meirisa Alnaz[3]

1 Faculty of Medicine, Division of Pediatric Surgery, Department of Surgery, Universitas Sumatera Utara, Medan, Indonesia

2 Faculty of Medicine, Universitas Sumatera Utara, Medan, Indonesia

3 Faculty of Medicine, Division of Pediatric Surgery, Department of Surgery, Universitas Padjajaran, Bandung, Indonesia

*Address all correspondence to: binnazief@gmail.com

IntechOpen

© 2022 The Author(s). Licensee IntechOpen. This chapter is distributed under the terms of the Creative Commons Attribution License (http://creativecommons.org/licenses/by/3.0), which permits unrestricted use, distribution, and reproduction in any medium, provided the original work is properly cited.

References

[1] Almaymoof A, Hamawendi M. Acute appendicitis in children. Basrah: Lambert Academic Publishing; 2017

[2] Yang KT, Wei JCC, Chang R, Lin CC, Chen HH. Association between appendicitis and incident systemic sclerosis. Journal of Clinical Medicine. 2021;**10**:1-9

[3] Téoule P, de Laffolie J, Rolle U, Reißfelder C. Acute appendicitis in childhood and adolescence-an everyday clinical challenge. Deutsches Ärzteblatt International. 2020;**117**:764-774

[4] di Saverio S, Podda M, de Simone B, Ceresoli M, Augustin G, Gori A, et al. Diagnosis and treatment of acute appendicitis: 2020 update of the WSES Jerusalem guidelines. World Journal of Emergency Surgery. 2020;**15**:1-42

[5] Wagner M, Tubre DJ, Asensio JA. Evolution and current trends in the management of acute appendicitis. Surgical Clinics of North America. 2018;**98**:1005-1023

[6] Drake RL, Vogl AW, Mitchell AWM. Gray's Anatomy for Students. 2nd ed. Philadelphia, PA: Curchill Livingstone; 2010

[7] Gilroy AM, Macpherson BR, Wikenheiser JC. Atlas of Anatomy. 4th ed. New York, NY: Thieme Publishers; 2020

[8] Hashmi S, Khattab A, Ehrenpreis ED. Physiology of the mesenteric circulation. In: The Mesenteric Organ in Health and Disease. Seattle, WA: Springer; 2021. pp. 107-119

[9] Moore KL, Dalley AF, Agur AMR. Moore Clinically Oriented Anatomy. 7th ed. Philadelphia, PA: Wolters Kluwer; 2014

[10] Girard-Madoux MJH, Gomez de Agüero M, Ganal-Vonarburg SC, Mooser C, Belz GT, Macpherson AJ, et al. The immunological functions of the appendix: An example of redundancy? Seminars in Immunology. 2018;**36**:31-44

[11] Di Saverio S, Birindelli A, Kelly MD, Catena F, Weber DG, Sartelli M, et al. WSES Jerusalem guidelines for diagnosis and treatment of acute appendicitis. World Journal of Emergency Surgery. 2016;**11**:1-25

[12] Stringer MD. Acute appendicitis. Journal of Paediatrics and Child Health. 2017;**53**:1071-1076

[13] Krzyzak M, Mulrooney SM. Acute appendicitis review: Background, epidemiology, diagnosis, and treatment. Cureus. 2020;**12**:10-15

[14] Becker P, Fichtner-Feigl S, Schilling D. Clinical management of appendicitis. Visceral Medicine. 2018;**34**:453-458

[15] Kooij IA, Sahami S, Meijer SL, Buskens CJ, te Velde AA. The immunology of the vermiform appendix: A review of the literature. Clinical and Experimental Immunology. 2016;**186**:1-9

[16] Jones MW, Lopez RA, Deppen JG. Appendicitis. Tampa Bay: StatPearls; 2022

[17] Mescher AL. Junqueira's Basic Histology Text and Atlas. 15th ed. New York, NY: McGraw-Hill; 2018

[18] López JJ, Deans KJ, Minneci PC. Nonoperative management of

appendicitis in children. Current Opinion in Pediatrics. 2017;**29**:358-362

[19] Mak GZ, Loeff DS. Paradigm shifts in the treatment of appendicitis. Pediatric Annals. 2016;**45**:e235-e240

[20] Petroianu A, Vinicius Villar Barroso T. Pathophysiology of acute appendicitis. Journal of Science Medical Gastroenterology and Hepatology. 2016;**4**(3):1062

[21] Solberg A, Holmdahl L, Falk P, Willén R, Palmgren I, Ivarsson ML. Tissue proteolysis in appendicitis with perforation. Journal of Surgical Research. 2011;**169**:194-201

[22] Perez KS, Allen SR. Complicated appendicitis and considerations for interval appendectomy. Jjournal of the American Academy of Physician Assistants. 2018;**31**:35-41

[23] Calgary Guide. Appendicitis: Pathogenesis and Clinical Findings. Calgary: Calgary Guide; 2022

[24] Simonetto DA, Singal AK, Garcia-Tsao G, Caldwell SH, Ahn J, Kamath PS. ACG clinical guideline: Disorders of the hepatic and mesenteric circulation. American Journal of Gastroenterology. 2020;**115**:18-40

[25] Baird DLH, Simillis C, Kontovounisios C, Rasheed S, Tekkis PP. Acute appendicitis. BMJ. 2017;**357**:j1703

[26] Cheluvappa R, Eri R, Luo AS, Grimm MC. Endothelin and vascular remodelling in colitis pathogenesis—appendicitis and appendectomy limit colitis by suppressing endothelin pathways. International Journal of Colorectal Disease. 2014;**29**:1321-1328

[27] de Costa. The appendix-mucosal immunity and tolerance in the gut: Consequences for the syndromes of appendicitis and its epidemiology. ANZ Journal of Surgery. 2022;**92**(4):653-660

[28] Fikri E, Nadjib Dahlan Lubis HM, Surya B, Siregar KB. The role of vascular endothelial growth factor as a predictor of complicated appendicitis in animal model oryctolagus cuniculus. Open Access Macedonian Journal of Medical Sciences. 2020;**8**:261-265

[29] Fikri E, Eyanoer PC. The determination of appendicitis from folate acid and vascular endothelial growth factor level in animal model: A review. Open Access Macedonian Journal of Medical Sciences. 2021;**9**:395-398

[30] Wilms IM, de Hoog DE, de Visser DC, Janzing HM. Appendectomy versus antibiotic treatment for acute appendicitis. Cochrane Database of Systematic Reviews. 9 Nov 2011;(11):CD008359. DOI: 10.1002/14651858.CD008359.pub2

[31] Apte RS, Chen DS, Ferrara N. VEGF in signaling and disease: Beyond discovery and development. Cell. 2019;**176**:1248-1264. DOI: 10.1016/j.cell.2019.01.021

[32] Shaik-Dasthagirisaheb YB, Varvara G, Murmura G, Saggini A, Potalivo G, Caraffa A, et al. Vascular endothelial growth factor (VEGF), mast cells and inflammation. International Journal of Immunopathology and Pharmacology. 2013;**26**:327-335

[33] van Le TH, Kwon SM. Vascular endothelial growth factor biology and its potential as a therapeutic target in rheumatic diseases. International Journal of Molecular Sciences. 2021;**22**(10):5387

[34] Pandey AK, Singhi EK, Arroyo JP, Ikizler TA, Gould ER, Brown J, et al. Mechanisms of VEGF (vascular

endothelial growth factor) inhibitor-associated hypertension and vascular disease. Hypertension. 2018;**71**:E1-E8

[35] Kokkonen TS, Karttunen TJ. Endothelial Fas-Ligand in Inflammatory Bowel Diseases and in Acute Appendicitis. Journal of Histochemistry and Cytochemistry. 2015;**63**:931-942

[36] Nurafni F, Fikri E, Surgeon P, Eyanoer PC. Folate acid analysis in predicting complicated appendicitis in animal model oryctolagus cuniculus. Pravara Medical Review. 2020;**12**:8-15